THE 400-CALORIE
MEDITERRANEAN
DIET COOKBOOK

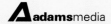

Adams Media
An Imprint of Simon & Schuster, Inc.
100 Technology Center Drive
Stoughton, Massachusetts 02072

First Adams Media trade paperback edition September 2021

ADAMS MEDIA and colophon are trademarks of Simon & Schuster.

For information about special discounts for bulk purchases, please contact Simon & Schuster Special Sales at 1-866-506-1949 or business@simonandschuster.com.

The Simon & Schuster Speakers Bureau can bring authors to your live event. For more information or to book an event contact the Simon & Schuster Speakers Bureau at 1-866-248-3049 or visit our website at www.simonspeakers.com.

Interior design by Priscilla Yuen
Photographs by Kelly Jaggers
Interior images © 123RF/9dreamstudio, Alfio Scisetti, Baiba Opule, tobi; Getty Images/Aamulya

Manufactured in the United States of America

1 2021

Library of Congress Cataloging-in-Publication Data
Names: Minaki, Peter, author.
Title: The 400-calorie Mediterranean diet cookbook / Peter Minaki.
Description: First Adams Media trade paperback edition. | Stoughton, MA: Adams Media, 2021. | Includes index.
Identifiers: LCCN 2021018952
| ISBN 9781507216736 (pb)
| ISBN 9781507216743 (ebook)
Subjects: LCSH: Cooking, Mediterranean. | Reducing diets. | LCGFT: Cookbooks.
Classification: LCC TX725.M35 M54 2021
| DDC 641.59/1822--dc23
LC record available at https://lccn.loc.gov/2021018952

ISBN 978-1-5072-1673-6
ISBN 978-1-5072-1674-3 (ebook)

Contains material adapted from the following titles published by Adams Media, an Imprint of Simon & Schuster, Inc.: *The Everything® Mediterranean Diet Book* by Connie Diekman, MEd, RD, LD, FADA, and Sam Sotiropoulos, copyright © 2010, ISBN 978-1-4405-0674-1; *The Everything® Mediterranean Cookbook, 2nd Edition* by Peter Minaki, copyright © 2013, ISBN 978-1-4405-6855-8; and *The Everything® Healthy Mediterranean Cookbook* by Peter Minaki, copyright © 2019, ISBN 978-1-5072-1150-2.

THE 400-CALORIE MEDITERRANEAN DIET COOKBOOK

100 Recipes under 400 Calories— for Easy and Healthy Weight Loss!

PETER MINAKI

ADAMS MEDIA

New York London Toronto Sydney New Delhi

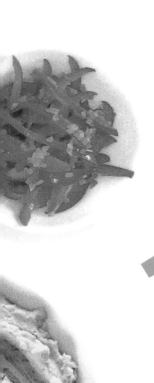

CONTENTS

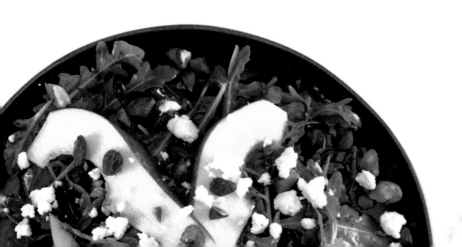

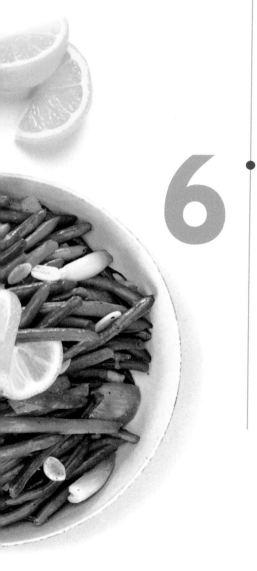

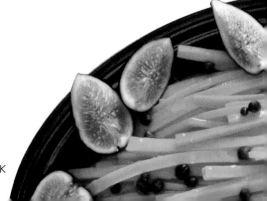

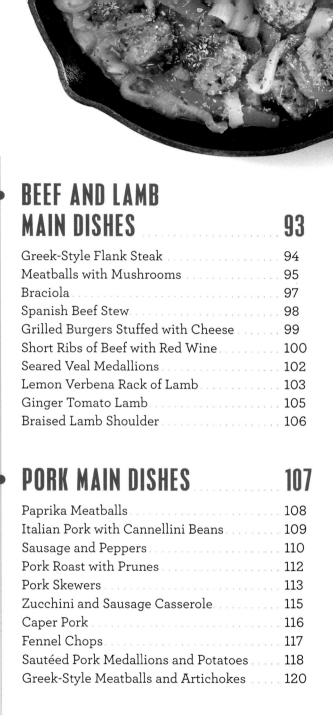

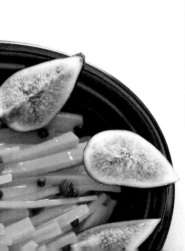

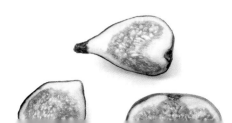

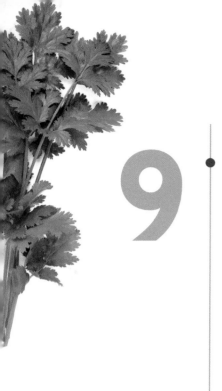

11

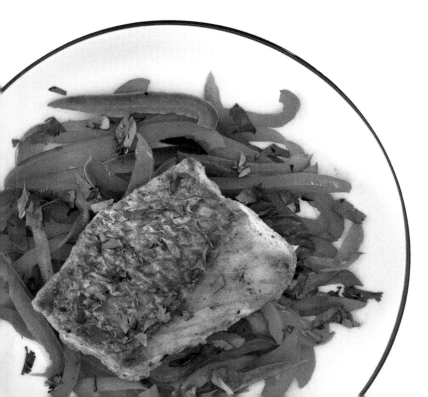

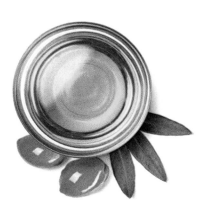

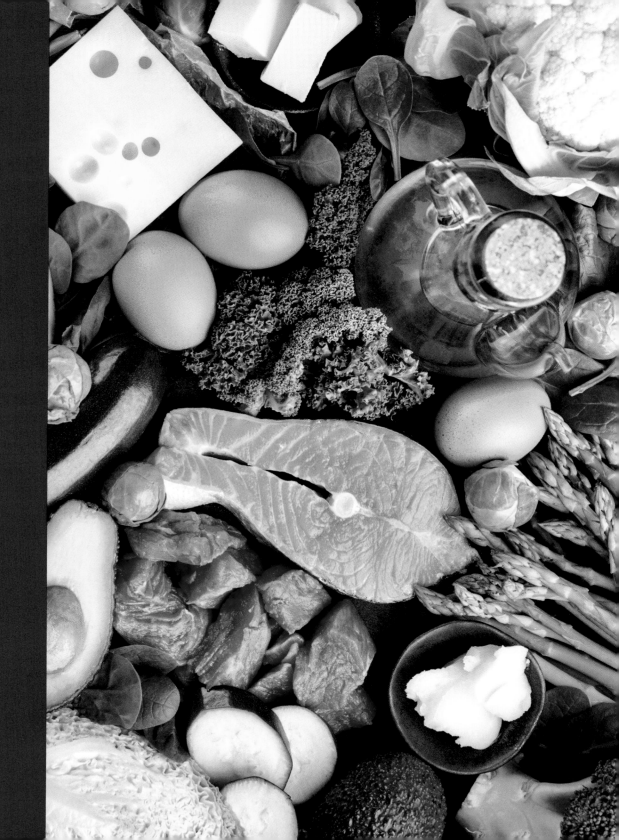

INTRODUCTION

Just because you're counting calories doesn't mean your food has to be bland, boring, or repetitive. Instead, enjoy distinctively savory and sweet flavors without leaving your kitchen by adopting the Mediterranean diet!

The diet of many people in the Mediterranean region includes high-quality protein sources, healthy fats, and naturally low-calorie dishes. No matter where you live, you can adopt this lifestyle of healthy eating and regular exercise to enjoy its many benefits—including weight loss.

Throughout this book, you'll find one hundred recipes with fewer than 400 calories per serving that are flavorful, nutrient-rich, and good for your overall health. With recipes ranging from Tomato and Goat Cheese Breakfast Casserole for breakfast to Oven-Poached Bass with Kalamata Chutney for dinner to Berries and Meringue for dessert, you'll find that cooking low-calorie dishes can be easy, fun, and delicious. The recipes use ingredients that you can find easily at local grocery stores, making them a snap to assemble. Plus, you'll be reaping the other benefits of Mediterranean cooking, such as a lower risk of heart disease and cancer, reduced inflammation, and the potential to control diabetes. You'll also learn how to incorporate exercise into your life to complement the healthy diet and keep your body strong and fit.

Whether you're following a 1,200- or 1,500-calorie diet or just trying to keep an eye on your daily calorie intake, these recipes will help you feel full morning, noon, and night. It's not just the calorie count that makes these recipes stand out; they're also packed with key vitamins and minerals as well. For example, you'll enjoy heart-healthy fiber from sesame seeds; antioxidants from olive oil; protein, selenium, and vitamin B_6 from sea bass; and bone-strengthening calcium from feta cheese.

These simple, low-calorie meals are easy to whip up, but satisfying and delicious enough for even the most sophisticated palates. Imagine yourself enjoying the brilliant sunshine and sea breezes of the Mediterranean while you indulge in these mouthwatering recipes!

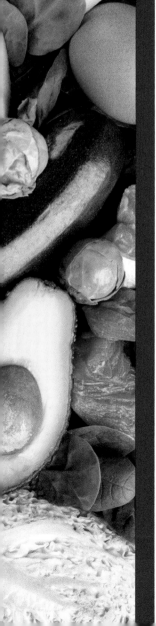

CHAPTER 1

Lose Weight with the Mediterranean Diet

If you're looking to lose weight, the Mediterranean diet is a great choice. Of course, there are many different cultures within the Mediterranean region, but in general, the people in this area eat very flavorful, low-calorie foods and don't treat any nutrients as "off limits." This all-encompassing approach means you'll find the diet easier to adopt—and maintain over the long term. Combining the nutrient-rich but naturally low-calorie foods of this region with regular exercise will help you lose weight in a sustainable way. The one hundred recipes in this book are 400 calories or fewer, and offer a variety of flavor profiles and easy-to-track calorie counts. In this chapter, you'll learn how embracing the Mediterranean region's approach to eating and movement can help you get to—and stay at—the weight you want.

FACTORS THAT CONTRIBUTE TO YOUR WEIGHT

According to the National Center for Health Statistics (part of the US Centers for Disease Control and Prevention), more than 73 percent of Americans are overweight or obese. Many people want to lose weight, but find it difficult to follow popular fad diets that often severely restrict certain nutrients. Plus, for many people, the cause of their excess weight is multifaceted: low levels of activity, portion sizes that are too large, and too many foods that lack nutrients. In order to lose weight, all of those issues must be addressed.

NUTRIENT-RICH FOODS

Nutrient-rich foods provide substantial amounts of vitamins and minerals and relatively few calories. Eating nutrient-rich foods like whole fruits and vegetables, healthy oils, whole grains, and protein provide your body with the energy you need without excess calories. On the other hand, foods with "empty calories" contain more calories and fewer vitamins and minerals than you need.

HOW THE MEDITERRANEAN DIET CAN HELP YOU LOSE WEIGHT

The Mediterranean diet can be a good option for those wishing to lose weight because it offers a variety of foods; focuses more on low-calorie, high-fiber plant foods; and recognizes the importance of activity. Before you take up the Mediterranean diet for your weight-loss plan, let's look at what the science says about its role in weight loss.

CALORIES AND WEIGHT LOSS

The key to losing weight is to burn more calories than you consume. Eating a low-calorie diet and exercising regularly makes that process easier.

Many studies have shown that the Mediterranean diet can help prevent obesity. Why exactly does it work? Mainly because the diet provides most nutrients needed for health; it is high in fiber; the source of fat is of a healthier type; and more of the protein comes from plant foods. In addition, the Mediterranean diet offers a higher fat content, which can aid in satiety, making it easier to follow the diet. At the same time, the fiber content also keeps you feeling full longer, so it is easier to space meals further apart.

Another aspect of the Mediterranean diet, studied by several different researchers, is the role of fluid content in foods. Fruits and vegetables provide a lot of water, and as Dr. Barbara Rolls has shown, high volumes of water in the foods you consume aid feelings of fullness. In a study in the journal *Nutrición Hospitalaria*, authors Marta Garaulet and F. Pérez de Heredia reported that in addition to the benefits already listed, three other factors also make the Mediterranean diet a good choice for weight loss:

1 The diet has a relatively high-carbohydrate content, which helps avoid the triggers for hunger, thus reducing the frequency of binge eating.

2 The diet can be followed comfortably for long periods of time.

3 The diet is tastier than many low-fat diet options.

The Mayo Clinic released a study in 2020 that also emphasized the importance of eating fewer calories. This research showed that lower-calorie foods, smaller portion sizes, and exercise are key to sustainable weight management.

Sweets Aren't Off Limits

When you look at the diets of some Mediterranean countries, it is very clear that sweets can fit very nicely into their overall healthful eating plan. The reason these sweets fit into the traditional eating plans of these countries is twofold:

1 The people of the Mediterranean region traditionally have a better perspective on portions, with desserts generally being very small.

2 These foods are enjoyed after they consume fruits, vegetables, beans, and grains as opposed to cutting back on those foods in order to consume larger portions of dessert. Many of the treats even include fruits or nuts as part of the recipe.

This healthier perspective about sweets makes it easier for you to enjoy them but still meet your weight loss goals.

OTHER HEALTH BENEFITS OF THE MEDITERRANEAN DIET

In addition to the potential for weight loss, this lifestyle also offers many other health benefits, including a reduced risk of several age-related diseases believed to be driven by inflammation: improved heart health, improved cholesterol levels, a reduction of symptoms of acid reflux, and the potential to control or prevent diabetes. Researchers are even studying whether it can lengthen your life span!

INCORPORATING ACTIVITY INTO YOUR DAY

A key part of the Mediterranean diet is moving your body every day. You'll likely find that regular exercise actually gives you more energy and might even inspire you to eat healthier as well.

The Benefits of Exercise

Besides burning calories, regular activity provides the following benefits:

- Strengthens the heart, lungs, and blood vessels
- Helps improve your mental state
- Can help lower blood triglycerides and cholesterol
- Reduces body fat and preserves muscle
- Helps lower blood pressure
- Lowers blood sugar levels

Regular activity keeps your body working at its peak, which then improves your overall quality of life.

How Much Activity Do You Need?

Current guidelines recommend adults get at least 2 ½ hours of moderate-intensity activity every week. Moderate activity is defined as walking briskly, doing water aerobics, or riding a bike. Along with this activity, adults need to do muscle-strengthening activities two or more days a week. Muscle-strengthening activities include lifting weights, working with resistance bands, doing push-ups or sit-ups, or yoga. This activity should include all parts of the body, so make sure you work your arms, legs, back, chest, shoulders, and abdomen.

If you are able to do more vigorous activity, the guidelines call for 1 hour and 15 minutes of vigorous activity each week. Vigorous activities include jogging, running, swimming laps, riding a bike uphill, or playing tennis or other sports. In addition to vigorous activity, you should still do the muscle-strengthening activities each week.

> **TALK TO YOUR DOCTOR**
>
> Before you embark on any type of activity routine, make sure you get a physical and talk with your doctor about your plans. Discuss all types of activities you're considering to be sure you are fit for all of them.

Getting Started

If your current activity level is little to no activity, start slowly with 10 minutes each day—or even 10 minutes a couple days each week—and then add more time as your fitness develops. Increase the number of minutes you exercise when your activity becomes too easy and you aren't breathing as heavily as you did when you first started doing the routine. Set short-term goals and celebrate your success along the way. The goal with exercise is the length of time, so whether you aim for 150 minutes of moderate-intensity activity or 75 minutes of vigorous activity, the important thing is to get to that level and continue with that plan.

If you are new to lifting weights, you might want to take a class or work with a trainer to learn proper form. Overall, the goal with muscle strengthening is to do 8–12 repetitions of each lift, 2–3 times. It is always best to do one set and then do another activity before returning to do the second set. Muscles tire very quickly, so doing too many reps can cause muscles to tire and you won't be able to get as much benefit from lifting at that point.

BALANCE YOUR MUSCLE WORK

When lifting weight, it is a good idea to work opposing muscles so that muscle development is even. If you are doing an arm curl where you roll the weight into your body, make the next activity a press so that you extend your arms out from your body.

Taking Exercise to the Next Level

If you're in good shape, or if you want to lower your cholesterol more or keep your blood sugar low enough to avoid medication, try building up your activity goals. If you're striving for substantial health benefits, the Centers for Disease Control and Prevention recommends the following for adults:

▶ 5 hours or 300 minutes of moderate-intensity activity each week plus muscle strengthening

▶ 2 ½ hours or 150 minutes of vigorous activity each week plus muscle strengthening

▶ A blend of moderate and vigorous activity each week plus muscle strengthening

Again, always check with your doctor before you adopt or make a significant change to your workout regimen.

Eating Balanced Meals Before and After Exercise

Choosing the right foods before and after a workout will ensure that muscles repair and rebuild. Physical activity burns calories, but if you are trying to lose weight you won't want to overeat before or after your activity; you *will* want to be sure you consume the right foods for activity. Muscles grow when they are fed with fuel and nutrients for building. Planning meals or snacks that combine carbohydrates and protein is the best way to fuel your workouts.

Meals for Short Workouts

If you are just starting out and your workouts aren't very long, you won't need a lot of extra nutrition for your workouts and you won't have to be as focused on when you eat. The longer or more intense a workout, the more important it is to fuel in a timely manner. For those just starting out, simply make sure that your meals and snacks combine some protein and some carbohydrates. An example of a morning meal might include the following:

- ▶ 1 cup of cooked oatmeal
- ▶ 2 tablespoons chopped dried apricots and raisins
- ▶ 2 tablespoons chopped nuts
- ▶ 1 cup skim milk (used to prepare oatmeal)
- ▶ 1 slice whole-wheat toast
- ▶ 2 teaspoons peanut butter (spread on toast)

If you plan to work out first thing in the morning, you may not want to eat a big meal first, so consider grabbing something small like a piece of fruit with a touch of peanut butter; if you plan to work out for only 30 minutes, a piece of fruit might be enough.

Meals for Longer Workouts

As your workouts reach 30–40 minutes, you will need to think about what to eat after a workout to replace the energy you used and allow your muscles to repair and grow. Remember that if you are trying to lose or maintain weight, you need to keep calories and portions in mind.

TIMING MATTERS TOO

For the best repair and development of your muscles, refuel with some protein and carbohydrates within 2 hours of working your muscles. With this in mind, try to plan your heavy workouts 3–4 hours after a large meal so you don't get stomach cramps from having just consumed a meal. This also means that right after your workout you can have another meal, thus scheduling your hunger and your muscle-fueling needs together.

Working In High-Fiber Foods at the Right Time

The Mediterranean diet is built around beans, whole grains, fruits, and vegetables, which all provide lots of fiber. While fiber is a plus to overall health and satiety, it can impact how you feel during physical activity. High-fiber foods require more time to digest—that is why they help you feel full longer—but if you exercise too soon after a meal, this extra digestion time can lead to stomach cramping. You may need to consume higher-fiber foods earlier in your day, well before your activity.

In addition to needing more time for digestion, high-fiber foods require extra fluid intake. If you plan to work out after a meal that is high in fiber, you might need to boost your fluid intake to stay hydrated during your workout.

Hydration needs vary from individual to individual, but as a general rule, you need to consume 2 cups of fluid 2 hours before your activity, another cup 1 hour before, and 4–6 ounces of water or sports drink for every 15 minutes of activity during your workout.

KEEPING THE WEIGHT OFF

Making changes in your eating and activity habits takes time. Some research studies show that it can take between 90 and 120 days for a new behavior to become a habit, so be patient with yourself. Remember that healthy weight loss happens slowly, about one pound per week on average, so plan your goals with that in mind.

In addition to healthy weight loss happening slowly, it is not uncommon for weight loss to go through plateaus—periods where no weight loss occurs. Weight loss that represents changes in body fat is gradual, but with steady commitment to a long-term goal, you can make it through these plateaus.

Rewarding Yourself

Building in rewards for your efforts is one way to get through a plateau or celebrate a milestone. Try to make these rewards non-food-based if possible. For example, splurge on new workout gear if you have been faithfully following your workout plan or unwind with a cup of herbal tea after a day of healthy meals. Whatever you decide on for your rewards, make sure you savor them and feel proud of your progress.

FUELING YOUR WEIGHT LOSS

Now that you have some background on why the Mediterranean diet can help you with your weight loss goals, it's time to get cooking. Each recipe has a full nutritional panel so you can easily track your calorie intake and meet your daily goals. You can flip through this book page by page to decide which dishes you'll try, or jump right to a recipe you know you want to make first. Either way, you're sure to find meals that your whole family will enjoy!

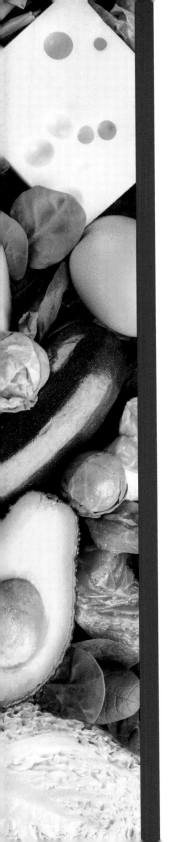

CHAPTER 2

Breakfast

It can be tempting to skip breakfast when you're counting calories, but studies show this is not a good choice for your body or mind. Instead, try the filling but naturally low-calorie dishes in this chapter to start your day on the right foot. Packed with fiber, protein, and vegetables, these recipes are both delicious and satisfying. Whether you are in the mood for a simple dish like Eggs in Italian Bread or a heartier option like Sausage Breakfast, you're sure to find something that fits into your schedule and nutritional plan.

Tomato and Goat Cheese Breakfast Casserole

Tomatoes and oregano pair elegantly with goat cheese to create a luscious casserole that works just as well on a midweek morning as it does for a weekend breakfast party. This decadent breakfast is high on flavor but low in calories!

SERVES 6

8 large eggs

1 cup whole milk

½ teaspoon salt

1 teaspoon freshly ground black pepper

2 cups cherry tomatoes, halved

¼ cup fresh oregano, chopped

4 ounces goat cheese, diced

1 teaspoon olive oil

1. Whisk eggs, milk, salt, and pepper together in a medium bowl. Stir in tomatoes, oregano, and goat cheese and mix well.

2. Spray a 4- to 5-quart slow cooker with nonstick cooking spray. Pour egg mixture into slow cooker. Cover and cook on low 4–6 hours or on high 2–3 hours. The casserole is done when a knife inserted into the center comes out clean. Serve hot.

Calories 200

PER SERVING

Fat 13g
Sodium 400mg
Carbohydrates 6g
Fiber 1g
Sugar 3g
Protein 14g

Frittata

This Italian egg dish is like a quiche without a crust. It's a great way to use leftover potatoes and any vegetables in your refrigerator. The low-calorie bell peppers are packed with vitamin C, which can boost immunity.

SERVES 8

1 pound Idaho potatoes, peeled and thickly sliced

2 medium yellow bell peppers, seeded and sliced

2 medium red bell peppers, seeded and sliced

2 medium green bell peppers, seeded and sliced

1 large red onion, peeled and sliced

2 teaspoons extra-virgin olive oil

1 teaspoon salt, divided

1/2 teaspoon freshly ground black pepper, divided

3 large eggs

6 large egg whites

1 cup plain low-fat yogurt

1 cup whole milk

3 ounces grated fontina or Gouda cheese

1 tablespoon chopped fresh oregano leaves

1　Preheat oven to 375°F.

2　Toss potatoes, bell peppers, and onion in oil and place on a large baking sheet. Season with 1/2 teaspoon salt and 1/4 teaspoon black pepper. Roast for 10 minutes.

3　In a medium baking dish, add roasted vegetables in one layer.

4　In a medium bowl, whisk eggs, egg whites, yogurt, milk, cheese, and remaining 1/2 teaspoon salt and 1/4 teaspoon black pepper. Pour egg mixture into baking dish over vegetables.

5　Bake until eggs are completely set, about 30 minutes. Sprinkle with oregano and serve.

Calories 200

PER SERVING

Fat 8g
Sodium 490mg
Carbohydrates 21g
Fiber 3g
Sugar 7g
Protein 12g

FOR THE MEAT LOVER

If you want to boost the protein in this dish, consider adding chopped bacon, sausage, or ham to this recipe.

Eggs in Italian Bread

Use the best crusty bread you can find for a classic Italian breakfast. This simple but filling dish feels fancy but comes together in minutes.

SERVES 6

6 (2") slices crusty Italian bread

3 teaspoons olive oil, divided

2 medium red bell peppers, seeded and thinly sliced

1 small shallot, peeled and minced

6 large eggs

1/2 teaspoon salt

1/2 teaspoon freshly ground black pepper

1　Using a round cookie cutter or glass, cut out large circles from the center of each bread slice. Discard center pieces and set hollowed-out bread slices aside.

2　Heat 1 teaspoon oil in a medium skillet over medium heat. Sauteé bell peppers and shallot 5–7 minutes or until tender. Remove from skillet and place on a tray lined with paper towels to absorb excess oil; keep warm.

3　Heat remaining 2 teaspoons oil over medium-high heat in a large skillet. Place bread slices in pan. Crack one egg into hollowed-out center of each bread slice. Cook for 5 minutes, then flip carefully and cook for 3 minutes more. Transfer to plates and top with bell pepper mixture.

4　Season with salt and black pepper before serving.

Calories 160

PER SERVING

Fat 8g
Sodium 380mg
Carbohydrates 13g
Fiber 1g
Sugar 3g
Protein 9g

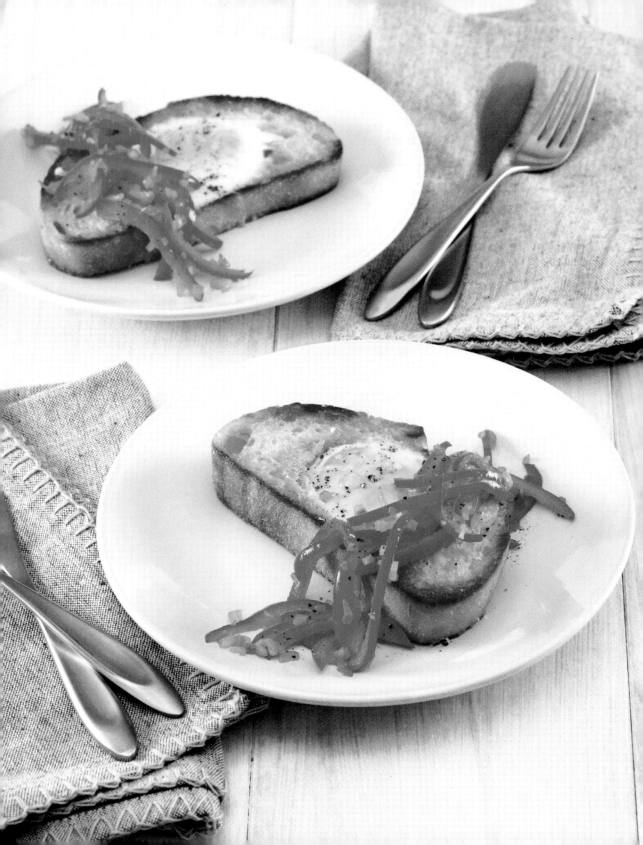

Baklava Oatmeal

If you've ever enjoyed baklava—sweet, nutty dessert bars found at many Greek restaurants—you're going to love this simple recipe. Baked with cinnamon and topped with a sweet baklava streusel and a drizzle of honey, this healthful oatmeal is a fiber-filled breakfast choice that will keep you full all morning.

SERVES 4

4 cups plus 1/2 teaspoon water, divided

1 cup steel-cut oats

1 1/2 teaspoons ground cinnamon, divided

1/2 cup chopped walnuts

1 teaspoon sugar

4 tablespoons honey

1. Spray the bottom of a small 1 1/2- to 3-quart slow cooker with nonstick cooking spray. Place 4 cups water, oats, and 1 teaspoon cinnamon in slow cooker. Stir until combined. Cover and cook on low 7–8 hours.

2. Just before serving, place walnuts in a large skillet over medium heat. Sprinkle with remaining 1/2 teaspoon cinnamon, sugar, and remaining 1/2 teaspoon water. Cook just until sugar begins to bubble and walnuts turn a light, toasted golden brown color.

3. Spoon walnut mixture over hot bowls of oatmeal. Drizzle with honey before serving.

Calories 320

PER SERVING

Fat 12g
Sodium 10mg
Carbohydrates 48g
Fiber 6g
Sugar 20g
Protein 7g

ABOUT STEEL-CUT OATS

Steel-cut oats are the whole-grain inner parts of the oat kernel that have been cut into pieces. They generally take longer to cook than traditional rolled oats, so preparing them overnight in a slow cooker is the perfect way to make them for breakfast the next day!

Raisin Bread

Start making this recipe the night before to enjoy fresh-baked bread the next morning.

SERVES 18

2 tablespoons active dry yeast

3½ cups lukewarm water

½ cup honey

1 teaspoon salt

¼ cup extra-virgin olive oil

3 tablespoons powdered milk

6¾ cups plus 3 tablespoons all-purpose flour, divided

1½ cups raisins

2 tablespoons coarse semolina flour

1 In a large bowl, mix yeast, water, and honey. Set for 7–10 minutes. Stir in salt, oil, and powdered milk. Gradually stir in 3 cups all-purpose flour. Stir in raisins and then gradually stir in another 3½ cups all-purpose flour. If the dough seems dry, add up to ½ cup water until it comes together. The dough should feel smooth and not too sticky.

2 Cover bowl with plastic wrap, but leave a small opening to allow the gases to escape. Let the dough rise in a cool place for a minimum of 6 hours or overnight.

3 When dough is ready, sprinkle ¼ cup of all-purpose flour on a work surface. Divide the dough in thirds and work with one piece at a time. Shape the dough into three oval loaves.

4 Sprinkle the semolina over a piece of parchment paper cut to the same size as a pizza stone or baking sheet. Place the loaves on the parchment, leaving room to allow dough to rise. Sprinkle remaining 3 tablespoons all-purpose flour over loaves. Let rise for 1½ hours. When loaves have risen, use a sharp knife to cut three shallow slices into the top of each loaf.

5 Preheat oven to 425°F. Set a pizza stone or large baking sheet on the middle rack to preheat. Add hot water to a broiler pan and place it on the top rack. Transfer loaves to the pizza stone or baking sheet and bake for 30–35 minutes until bread is golden. Carefully remove loaves from the oven and allow them to cool to room temperature before serving.

Calories 280

PER SERVING

Fat 3.5g
Sodium 135mg
Carbohydrates 57g
Fiber 2g
Sugar 16g
Protein 6g

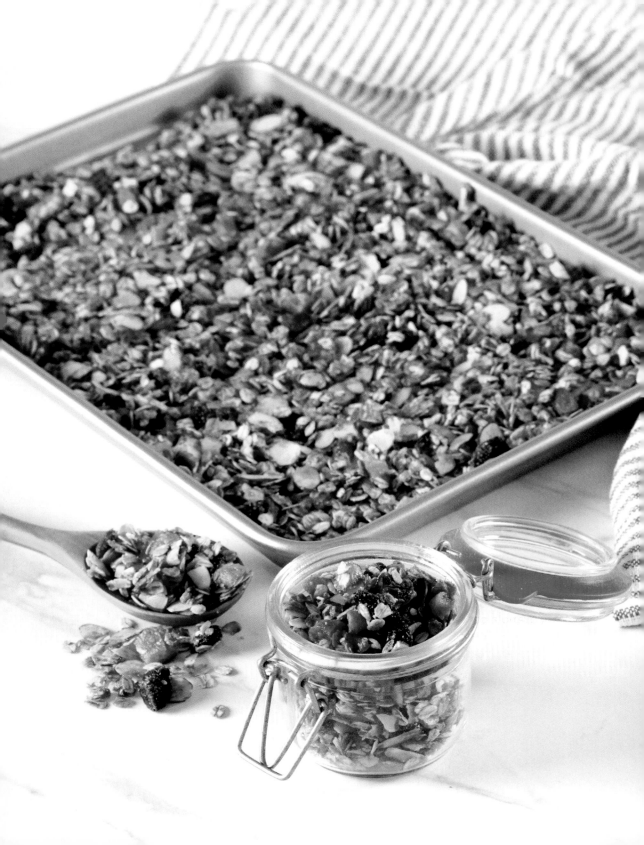

Fig, Apricot, and Almond Granola

Start your day with this energy-packed dish of oats with a hit of sweetness. Cardamom is a wonderful earthy spice that lends a citrusy note to this granola, while the figs make the dish sweet without adding processed sugar.

SERVES 16

1/3 cup vegetable oil	4 cups old-fashioned oats	1/2 cup packed brown sugar
1/3 cup honey	1 1/4 cups sliced almonds	1/2 teaspoon salt
2 tablespoons sugar	1/2 cup chopped dried apricots	1/2 teaspoon ground cardamom
1 teaspoon vanilla extract	1/2 cup chopped dried figs	

1. Preheat oven to 300°F. Lightly spray two large baking sheets with nonstick cooking spray.

2. In a small saucepan over medium heat, add vegetable oil, honey, granulated sugar, and vanilla. Cook for 5 minutes or until sugar is dissolved. Remove pan from heat and cool for 2 minutes.

3. In a large bowl, combine oats, almonds, apricots, figs, brown sugar, salt, and cardamom. Mix with your hands to combine.

4. Pour honey mixture over oat mixture. Using your hands (if it is too hot, use a wooden spoon), toss ingredients together to make sure everything is well coated. Line two medium baking sheets with parchment paper or spray with nonstick cooking spray. Spread granola evenly over sheets. Bake 30 minutes, stirring every 10 minutes.

5. Let granola cool completely on the baking sheets then break it up into pieces before serving. Store in an airtight container up to three weeks.

Calories 250

PER SERVING

Fat 10g
Sodium 75mg
Carbohydrates 37g
Fiber 4g
Sugar 17g
Protein 5g

DRIED FRUITS

Dried fruits such as figs, raisins, dates, and apricots have been part of the Mediterranean diet for centuries. Drying fruit is one of the oldest forms of preservation and is still popular today.

Breakfast Risotto

The creamy heartiness of risotto isn't just for dinner! Serve this breakfast variety as you would cooked oatmeal: topped with additional brown sugar, raisins or other dried fruit, and milk. A single portion will keep you full for hours.

SERVES 8

4 tablespoons unsalted butter, melted

1½ cups Arborio rice

3 small apples, peeled, cored, and sliced

1½ teaspoons ground cinnamon

⅛ teaspoon ground nutmeg

⅛ teaspoon ground cloves

⅛ teaspoon salt

⅓ cup packed light brown sugar

1 cup apple juice

3 cups whole milk

1. Spray a 4- to 5-quart slow cooker with nonstick cooking spray. Add butter and rice and stir to coat.

2. Add apples, cinnamon, nutmeg, cloves, salt, brown sugar, apple juice, and milk to slow cooker and stir to combine. Cover and cook on low 6–7 hours or on high 2–3 hours until rice is cooked through and is firm but not mushy. Serve immediately.

Calories 310

PER SERVING

Fat 9g
Sodium 80mg
Carbohydrates 52g
Fiber 3g
Sugar 21g
Protein 6g

Greek Biscotti

These crunchy cookies (sometimes called paximadia) are a wonderful accompaniment to your morning coffee. The combination of almond and orange offers a distinct flavor profile that will help wake you up.

SERVES 36

¼ cup fresh orange juice	1½ teaspoons ground cinnamon	1½ tablespoons baking powder
1 tablespoon grated orange zest	¼ teaspoon ground cloves	1 cup chopped almonds
¾ cup vegetable oil	¾ cup sugar	3 cups all-purpose flour
½ cup dry white wine	¼ teaspoon baking soda	1 cup sesame seeds

1. Preheat oven to 350°F. Add orange juice, orange zest, vegetable oil, wine, cinnamon, cloves, sugar, baking soda, and baking powder to a food processor and process until the ingredients are well incorporated. In a large bowl, stir almonds and flour together. Pour orange juice mixture into flour mixture. Use a wooden spoon to combine until a soft dough forms.

2. Divide dough and form three equal loaves (9" × 3"). Place equal amounts of sesame seeds on three pieces of wax paper. Wrap the paper around each loaf or roll the dough around on the paper so the sesame seeds coat the entire loaf. Repeat with the remaining loaves.

3. Place loaves on a large baking sheet lined with parchment paper. Bake on the middle rack for 20 minutes. Take baking sheet out of the oven and reduce temperature to 300°F.

4. Cool loaves for 2 minutes. Slice each loaf along its width into ¾" slices with a serrated knife. Lay the slices flat on the baking sheet, and bake for 10 minutes more. Turn off the oven, but leave biscotti in the oven for 30 minutes more.

5. Serve immediately or store biscotti in a sealed container for up to six months.

Calories 130

PER SERVING

Fat 8g
Sodium 15mg
Carbohydrates 14g
Fiber 1g
Sugar 4g
Protein 2g

Sausage Breakfast

This hearty breakfast is infused with Spanish flavors. The traditional sausage for this dish is a smoky chorizo, but you can use your favorite type, including a chicken variety. You can also switch up the types of vegetables and cheese as well depending on your preferences and what you have on hand.

SERVES 8

8 ounces chorizo, diced

1/4 cup water

3 large potatoes, peeled and diced

1 large onion, peeled and sliced

1 large green bell pepper, seeded and sliced

1 large red bell pepper, seeded and sliced

1 teaspoon smoked paprika

1/2 teaspoon freshly ground black pepper

1/2 teaspoon fresh thyme leaves

3/4 teaspoon salt, divided

1 cup grated graviera or Gruyère cheese

3 tablespoons extra-virgin olive oil, divided

8 large eggs

1 In a large skillet over medium-high heat, add sausage and water. Sauté for 3 minutes or until water evaporates and sausage is crispy. Add potatoes and stir to coat in the sausage drippings. Reduce heat to medium and cook for 5 minutes more.

2 Add onion, bell peppers, and smoked paprika. Cook for 3 minutes more. Season with black pepper, thyme, and 1/2 teaspoon salt. Reduce heat to medium-low and cook for 10–15 minutes or until potatoes are fork-tender. Sprinkle with cheese and take skillet off heat. The residual heat will melt the cheese.

3 In another large skillet, add 2 tablespoons oil and fry each egg to your liking (sunny-side up or over easy). Season eggs with remaining 1/4 teaspoon salt.

4 To serve, place a scoop of sausage and onion mixture onto each plate and a fried egg on top. Drizzle with remaining 1 tablespoon oil. Serve hot.

Calories 370

PER SERVING

Fat 24g
Sodium 790mg
Carbohydrates 20g
Fiber 1g
Sugar 3g
Protein 21g

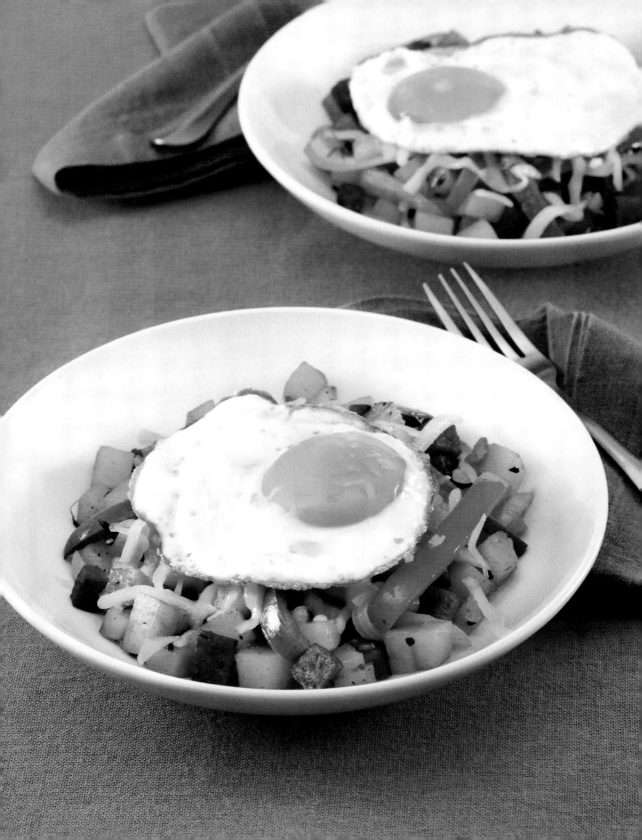

Homemade Greek Yogurt

*Greeks have been making and consuming yogurt for thousands of years,
and now Greek-style yogurt is available in most US grocery stores too.
Store-bought varieties sometimes have a good amount of added sugar,
though, so try this homemade version and mix in fresh fruit instead.*

SERVES 32

16 cups whole milk   ½ cup plain full-fat yogurt (containing active live cultures)

---

1 Preheat oven to 200°F. In a large pot over medium-high heat, add milk and bring to a boil. Reduce heat to medium-low and simmer for 15 minutes, and then take pot off heat. Do not cover pot.

2 Using a candy thermometer, allow milk to cool to 110°F–115°F. When you have reached the desired temperature, add ½ cup of warmed milk with yogurt in a small bowl. Stir to combine. Add milk and yogurt back to the pot and stir to combine.

3 Turn off the oven. Ladle milk-yogurt mixture into storage containers (plastic containers are okay because the oven is at a low temperature) and place on a baking tray in the oven. The yogurt will set in 8–12 hours (check it after 8 hours).

4 Refrigerate yogurt for at least 4 hours, but preferably overnight, before serving. This yogurt will keep in the refrigerator for up to two weeks.

Calories 80

PER SERVING

Fat 4g
Sodium 55mg
Carbohydrates 6g
Fiber 0g
Sugar 6g
Protein 4g

WHY YOU SHOULD EAT MORE YOGURT

Yogurt is easier to digest than milk, and it contributes to good colon health. This immunity booster is high in protein and rich in calcium, and aids in the absorption of B vitamins. Eat yogurt every day!

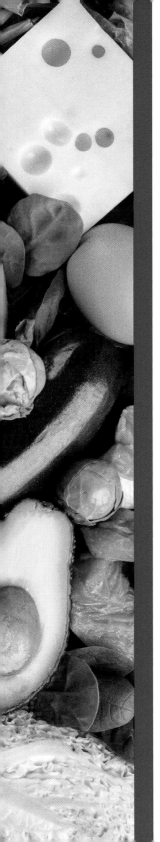

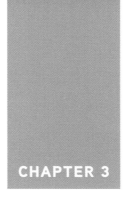

CHAPTER 3

Soups and Salads

Whether you want an appetizer or a light lunch, soups and salads are great options. The recipes in this chapter use fresh fruits and vegetables and flavorful spices to give each dish a unique flavor. Try the Spinach Salad with Apples and Mint on a hot day or the warm Italian Wedding Soup on a cold day; this chapter offers a variety of options.

Dandelion and White Bean Soup

Dandelion greens have a hearty, earthy flavor similar to radicchio or endive. The seasonings and fresh ingredients in this salad give it a lot of flavor without a lot of calories!

SERVES 6

1 teaspoon extra-virgin olive oil

2 medium onions, peeled and chopped

3 medium carrots, peeled and chopped

3 stalks celery, ends trimmed and chopped

4 cloves garlic, peeled and minced

8 cups vegetable stock

1 bay leaf

1/4 cup chopped fresh parsley

2 teaspoons fresh thyme leaves

1 teaspoon salt

1/2 teaspoon freshly ground black pepper

2 cups fresh dandelion greens, steamed until wilted

1 cup cooked cannellini beans

1/4 cup grated Romano or Parmesan cheese

1. Heat oil in a large pot over medium heat for 30 seconds. Add the onions, carrots, celery, and garlic. Cook for 5 minutes or until vegetables soften.

2. Add stock, increase heat to medium-high, and bring soup to a boil. Reduce heat to medium and cook for 1½ hours.

3. Add bay leaf, parsley, thyme, salt, and pepper. Cook for 30 minutes. Add dandelion greens and beans. Cook for 15 minutes more. Remove bay leaf.

4. Serve soup with a sprinkle of cheese on top.

Calories 130

PER SERVING

Fat 2.5g
Sodium 610mg
Carbohydrates 21g
Fiber 5g
Sugar 7g
Protein 7g

DANDELION GREENS

Dandelions grow in the Mediterranean countryside. Many people forage for the young, tender plants in the spring when they are not too bitter. Try dandelion greens in your salads or boil them and toss them in a little olive oil and lemon juice.

Beet Soup

Beets are a nutritional powerhouse that contain fiber, iron, and vitamin C, and they're naturally low in calories. Consuming beets might even help lower blood pressure! To add some creaminess to this flavorful soup, add a dollop of strained Greek yogurt to each bowl.

SERVES 6

2 large beets

¼ cup plus 1 tablespoon extra-virgin olive oil, divided

3 medium onions, peeled and sliced

3 cloves garlic, peeled and smashed

2 medium carrots, peeled and sliced

2 stalks celery, ends trimmed and sliced

2 cups finely sliced white cabbage

1 cup tomato purée

½ cup chopped fresh parsley

7 cups beef stock

2 large potatoes, peeled and cut into cubes

2 teaspoons salt

½ teaspoon freshly ground black pepper

¼ cup red wine vinegar

½ cup chopped fresh dill

1 Preheat oven to 450°F. Rub beets with 1 tablespoon oil. Wrap them in aluminum foil and place on a baking sheet. Bake for 45 minutes or until fork-tender. Peel skins off beets with the back of a knife and discard. Chop beets into ½" chunks.

2 Heat remaining ¼ cup oil in a large pot over medium heat for 30 seconds. Add the onions, garlic, carrots, and celery, and cook for 15 minutes. Add cabbage, tomato purée, parsley, and beets. Cook for 5 minutes more.

3 Add stock and potatoes and increase heat to medium-high. Bring soup to a boil. Reduce heat to medium-low and cook for 45–60 minutes or until potatoes are cooked. Season with salt and pepper.

4 Stir in vinegar and dill and serve.

Calories 350

PER SERVING

Fat 13g
Sodium 1,070mg
Carbohydrates 43g
Fiber 7g
Sugar 13g
Protein 17g

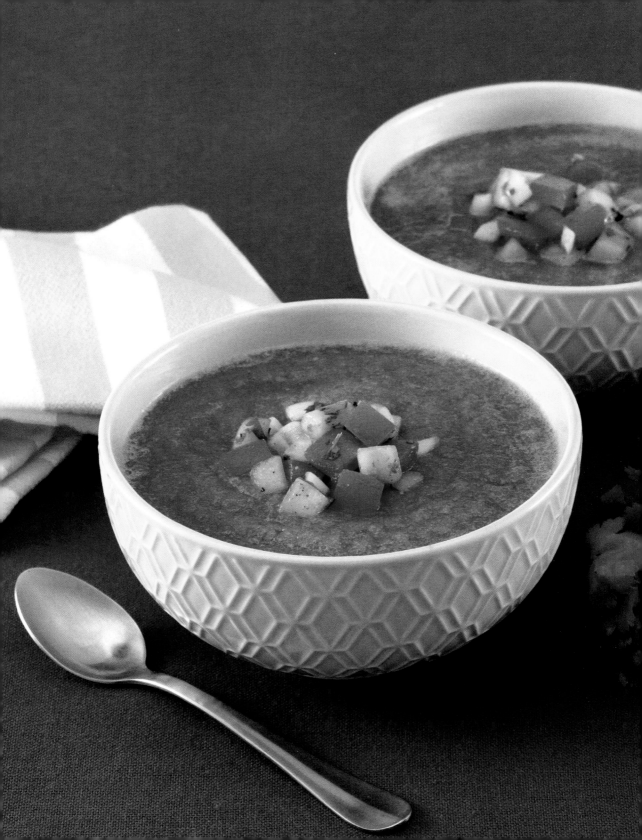

Gazpacho

This light but filling soup can really showcase your summer vegetable garden haul! Use only the freshest ingredients and remove the seeds from the vegetables. If you don't like cilantro, you can leave it out.

SERVES 6

2 large sweet onions, peeled and chopped

3 medium cucumbers, peeled and chopped

1½ pounds plum tomatoes, chopped

3 cloves garlic, peeled and minced

½ cup chopped fresh cilantro

1 chipotle pepper canned in adobo sauce, drained and chopped

2 tablespoons fresh lime juice

1½ teaspoons grated lime zest

¼ teaspoon hot pepper sauce

½ teaspoon freshly ground black pepper

1½ quarts vegetable broth

1. In a large bowl, mix together all ingredients except broth. Purée all but a quarter of mixture in a blender.

2. Add broth to puréed mixture in blender and continue to purée until smooth. To serve, ladle into serving bowls. Garnish with reserved vegetable mixture.

Calories 90

PER SERVING

Fat 0.5g
Sodium 570mg
Carbohydrates 19g
Fiber 3g
Sugar 12g
Protein 3g

Pumpkin Soup

In the summer, Mediterranean residents are all about zucchini, but in the winter months, pumpkin gets the spotlight. This comforting soup is perfect for those cold winter nights. Serve with a dollop of yogurt for a touch of creaminess.

SERVES 6

4 tablespoons unsalted butter

1 large onion, peeled and chopped

2 tablespoons grated ginger

2 cloves garlic, peeled and minced

8 cups vegetable stock

3 cups skinned, seeded, and chopped pumpkin

3 tablespoons chopped fresh parsley

2 teaspoons salt

$1/8$ teaspoon freshly ground black pepper

$1/8$ teaspoon ground nutmeg

$1/4$ cup chopped fresh chives

1. Melt butter in a large pot over medium heat. Add onion, ginger, and garlic. Reduce heat to medium, and cook for 5 minutes or until onion softens.

2. Add stock, pumpkin, and parsley. Increase heat to medium-high and bring soup to a boil. Reduce heat to medium-low, cover pot, and cook for 40–45 minutes. Season with salt, pepper, and nutmeg.

3. Use an immersion blender or a regular blender to carefully purée soup until smooth.

4. Stir in chives and serve.

Calories 120

PER SERVING

Fat 8g
Sodium 870mg
Carbohydrates 12g
Fiber 1g
Sugar 7g
Protein 2g

Italian Wedding Soup

This Italian classic is served at weddings or on other special occasions. If you make the meatballs ahead of time, you can prepare this soup on a weeknight in only 30 minutes! Feel free to add any leftover vegetables (like diced carrots) that you have in your fridge.

SERVES 6

3 slices Italian bread, toasted

3/4 pound lean ground beef

1 large egg, beaten

1 medium onion, peeled and chopped

3 cloves garlic, peeled and minced

1/4 cup chopped fresh parsley

1 tablespoon finely chopped fresh oregano

1 tablespoon finely chopped fresh basil

1 teaspoon salt

1/2 teaspoon freshly ground black pepper

1/2 cup grated Parmesan cheese, divided

8 cups chicken stock

1 cup roughly chopped fresh spinach, stems removed and steamed until wilted

---

1. Preheat oven to 375°F. Wet the toasted bread with water and then squeeze out all the liquid.

2. In a large bowl, combine bread, ground beef, egg, onion, garlic, parsley, oregano, basil, salt, pepper, and 1/4 cup Parmesan. Mix well. Form mixture into 1" meatballs and place on a large baking sheet lined with parchment paper. Bake for 20–30 minutes. Transfer meatballs to a tray lined with paper towels to absorb excess oil.

3. In a large pot over medium-high heat, bring stock to a boil and then reduce heat to medium-low. Add spinach and meatballs and cook for 30 minutes.

4. Ladle soup into serving bowls and sprinkle with remaining 1/4 cup Parmesan. Serve warm.

Calories 240

PER SERVING

Fat 12g
Sodium 740mg
Carbohydrates 12g
Fiber 1g
Sugar 2g
Protein 21g

Arugula, Pear, and Goat Cheese Salad

Arugula is a peppery salad green that is sometimes called "rocket" in grocery stores. This flavorful salad provides a lot of vitamin C and calcium too. This low-calorie lunch supplies a serving of both fruit and vegetables.

SERVES 6

2 medium pears, cored and cut into wedges

2 tablespoons fresh lemon juice, divided

1 tablespoon balsamic vinegar

1/3 cup extra-virgin olive oil

1/4 cup chopped fresh chives

1/2 teaspoon salt

1/8 teaspoon freshly ground black pepper

5 ounces baby arugula leaves

1/2 cup chopped unsalted pistachios

1/2 cup crumbled goat cheese

1. In a small bowl, toss pears with 1 tablespoon lemon juice.

2. In a large bowl, whisk remaining 1 tablespoon lemon juice, vinegar, oil, chives, salt, and pepper.

3. Add arugula to the bowl and toss to coat. Transfer to a serving platter.

4. Arrange pears over arugula and sprinkle with pistachios and cheese. Serve immediately.

Calories 240

PER SERVING

Fat 20g
Sodium 250mg
Carbohydrates 14g
Fiber 3g
Sugar 8g
Protein 5g

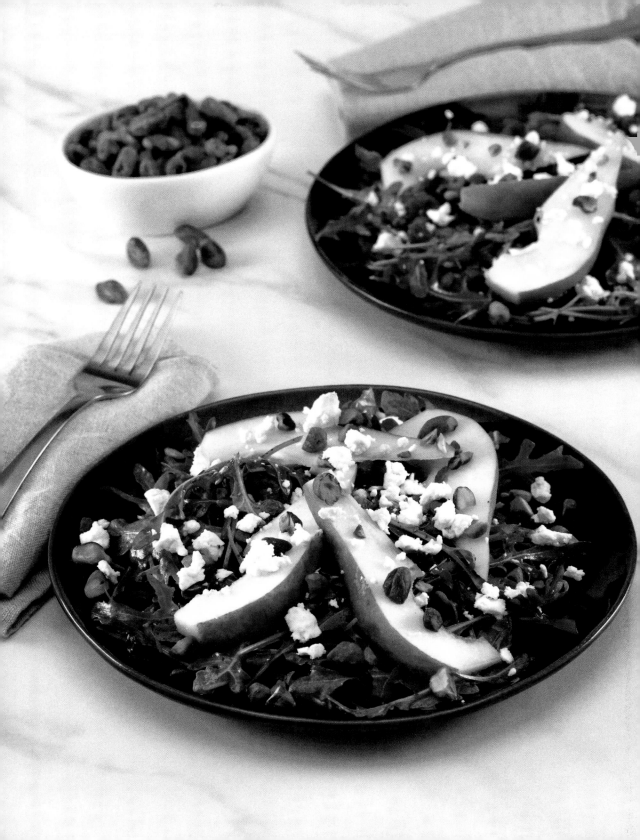

Artichoke Salad

Artichokes are high in fiber but low in fat, plus they contain vitamin C, vitamin K, and folate. Even better, a medium artichoke only contains about 70 calories! To add some protein, try topping this dish with fried calamari or grilled shrimp.

SERVES 8

2 medium onions, peeled and chopped, divided

1 medium carrot, peeled and diced, divided

1 tablespoon finely chopped celery

2 tablespoons fresh lemon juice

1 teaspoon salt

8 canned or jarred artichokes, rinsed and halved

1/2 cup extra-virgin olive oil, divided

1 medium red bell pepper, seeded and chopped

2 medium zucchini, ends trimmed and diced

1/2 cup fresh peas or thawed frozen peas

1 teaspoon salt

1/2 teaspoon freshly ground black pepper

10 pitted sliced Kalamata olives

1/4 cup finely chopped capers

1/2 cup chopped fresh mint

1. In a large deep skillet, add 3 inches of water and bring to a boil over medium-high heat. Add 2 tablespoons onions, 1 tablespoon carrots, celery, lemon juice, and salt. Return to a boil. Add artichokes and reduce heat to medium-low. Cook artichokes for 3 minutes or until tender. Remove artichokes with a slotted spoon, discard cooking liquid. Place artichokes in an ice bath to stop the cooking process. When artichokes have cooled, remove them from the ice bath and reserve.

2. Heat 1/4 cup oil in a large skillet over medium-high heat for 30 seconds. Add remaining onions, remaining carrots, and bell pepper. Reduce heat to medium and cook for 5–6 minutes. Add zucchini and cook for 2 minutes. Add peas and cook for 2 minutes more. Season with salt and black pepper. Remove from heat and allow vegetables to cool.

3. In a bowl, combine cooled vegetables, remaining 1/4 cup oil, olives, capers, and mint. Adjust seasoning with more salt and black pepper, if necessary.

4. Place 3–4 artichokes on each plate and top with vegetables. Serve salad at room temperature.

Calories 348

PER SERVING

Fat 27g
Sodium 1,266mg
Carbohydrates 24g
Fiber 5.5g
Sugar 8g
Protein 4g

Baby Greens with Chickpea Dressing

Puréed chickpeas are the base for this creamy, unusual salad dressing. Chickpeas are high in fiber, so they can improve your digestion and help with weight loss. Prewashed baby salad greens are easy to find at your local grocery store, so you can whip this up fresh for lunch in no time.

SERVES 6

¼ cup canned chickpeas, drained and rinsed

2 cloves garlic, peeled and minced

1 small shallot, peeled and minced

¼ cup chopped fresh parsley

½ teaspoon freshly ground black pepper

½ cup balsamic vinegar

¼ cup extra-virgin olive oil

5 ounces baby salad greens

1. In a food processor, purée chickpeas. Add garlic, shallot, parsley, pepper, and vinegar; pulse until well incorporated.

2. With processor running, slowly add oil and process until mixture emulsifies.

3. Place greens in a large salad bowl. Top with chickpea dressing and toss. Serve immediately.

Calories 120

PER SERVING

Fat 10g
Sodium 25mg
Carbohydrates 7g
Fiber 1g
Sugar 4g
Protein 1g

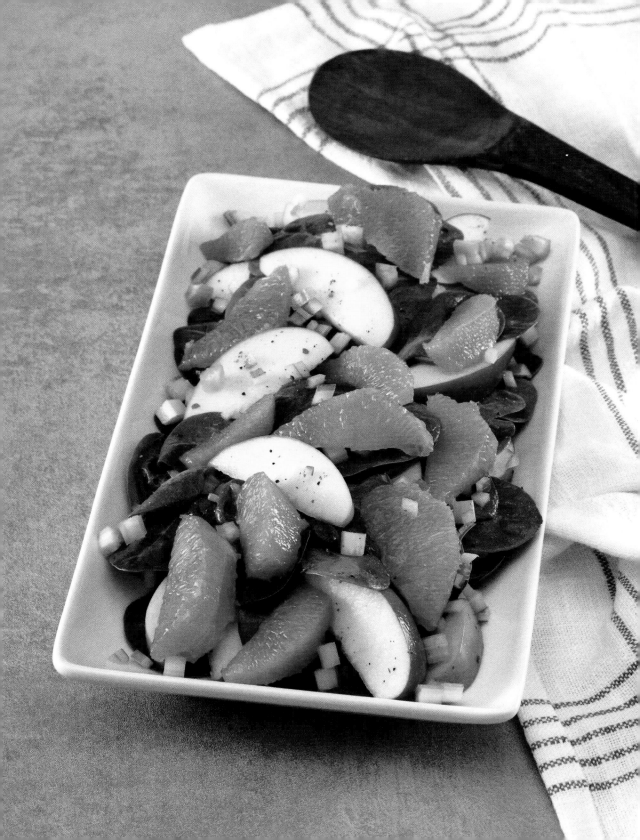

Spinach Salad with Apples and Mint

Use any variety of apples you like for this salad, but make sure you include at least one tart apple to balance out the flavors. Spinach is a nutritional powerhouse that provides vitamin C, vitamin K, calcium, and iron. Baby spinach is less tough than the regular variety, so it's perfect for eating raw in a salad.

SERVES 8

1/3 cup extra-virgin olive oil

10 fresh mint leaves, chopped

1 large orange, peeled and segmented, juice reserved

1 large grapefruit, peeled and segmented, juice reserved

1 tablespoon fresh lime juice

3/4 teaspoon salt

1/4 teaspoon freshly ground black pepper

1 large red apple, cored and sliced

1 large green apple, cored and sliced

1/3 cup finely chopped red onion

1 stalk celery, ends trimmed and chopped

5 ounces baby spinach

1. Process oil and mint in a food processor until well incorporated. Set aside and let mint infuse oil.

2. In a large bowl, whisk together reserved orange and grapefruit juices, lime juice, salt, pepper, and oil-mint infusion. Add apple slices, onion, and celery and toss to coat.

3. Add spinach and toss again to combine. Top salad with orange and grapefruit segments and serve.

Calories 150

PER SERVING

Fat 10g
Sodium 240mg
Carbohydrates 16g
Fiber 3g
Sugar 11g
Protein 1g

Strawberry and Feta Salad with Balsamic Dressing

This light salad is perfect when strawberries are in season. The sweet strawberries complement the tart and briny feta very well. You can make the dressing ahead of time, and store it in an airtight container in the refrigerator for several days.

SERVES 4

1 teaspoon Dijon mustard

3 tablespoons balsamic vinegar

1 clove garlic, peeled and minced

3/4 cup extra-virgin olive oil

1/2 teaspoon salt

1/8 teaspoon freshly ground black pepper

4 cups salad greens, rinsed and dried

1 pint ripe strawberries, hulled and halved

1 1/2 cups crumbled feta cheese

1. In a small bowl, whisk mustard, vinegar, garlic, oil, salt, and pepper to make the dressing.

2. In a large bowl, combine salad greens and dressing. Transfer to a serving platter and top with strawberries and feta.

3. Drizzle any remaining dressing over the salad and serve.

Calories 220

PER SERVING

Fat 18g
Sodium 500mg
Carbohydrates 10g
Fiber 2g
Sugar 6g
Protein 4g

IF IT'S NOT GREEK, IT'S NOT REAL FETA...

Greek feta cheese has a lower overall fat content and is more nutritionally beneficial than most other commercially available cheeses, including imitation cow's milk "feta" cheeses being produced and sold in North America and elsewhere.

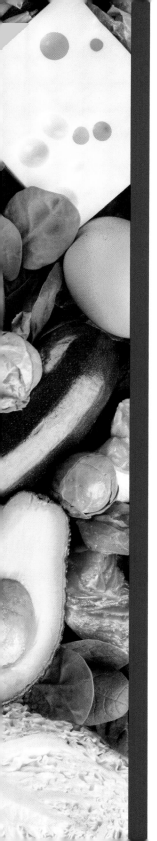

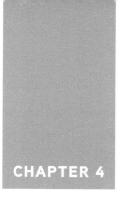

CHAPTER 4

Appetizers and Snacks

Whether you're planning a get-together with a dozen guests or just hanging out at home, appetizers can set the stage for a wonderful meal—or, when grouped together, even become a meal by themselves. The delicious bites in this chapter come from both the land and sea and won't fill you up too much. Best of all, since they're low in calories, you can indulge while staying on track with your daily calorie counts. Whether you try a savory dip like the Roasted Peppers, Eggplant, and Tomato Dip or a one-bite delight like the Phyllo-Wrapped Shrimp, you're sure to be transported to the Mediterranean region as you enjoy it.

Santorini's Yellow Pea Dip

Fava, in the Greek food sense, actually has nothing to do with fava beans. Rather, it's a dip made from yellow split peas. The yellow version of split peas has an earthier flavor than green split peas. Serve it with toasted pita bread or sturdy crackers.

SERVES 12

3 cups water

1 cup dried yellow split peas, rinsed

1/2 cup chopped onion

2 cloves garlic, peeled and smashed

2 bay leaves

1 teaspoon red wine vinegar

1/2 cup plus 1 tablespoon extra-virgin olive oil, divided

2 teaspoons fresh thyme leaves

1 teaspoon salt

1/2 teaspoon freshly ground black pepper

2 tablespoons thinly sliced red onion

1/2 teaspoon dried oregano

1. In a medium pot, combine water, peas, onion, garlic, and bay leaves over medium-high heat.

2. Cover pot and bring mixture to a boil. Reduce heat to medium-low and simmer for 15–20 minutes or until peas are tender.

3. Strain peas and remove bay leaves. Reserve a few whole peas for garnish. Combine pea mixture and vinegar in a food processor and process until mixture is smooth. With the processor running, slowly add 1/2 cup oil.

4. Remove dip from the processor and stir in thyme, salt, and pepper.

5. Garnish with reserved peas, red onion, and oregano. Drizzle with remaining 1 tablespoon oil. Serve warm or at room temperature.

Calories 160

PER SERVING

Fat 11g
Sodium 200mg
Carbohydrates 12g
Fiber 5g
Sugar 13g
Protein 4g

SPLIT PEAS: A NUTRITIONAL POWERHOUSE

Split peas are very high in dietary fiber and protein. They are an excellent and healthful alternative to meat proteins. Unlike other dried beans, you don't need to presoak them before cooking. Just give them a rinse and pick out any shriveled or broken peas, stones, or debris, and they are ready to cook.

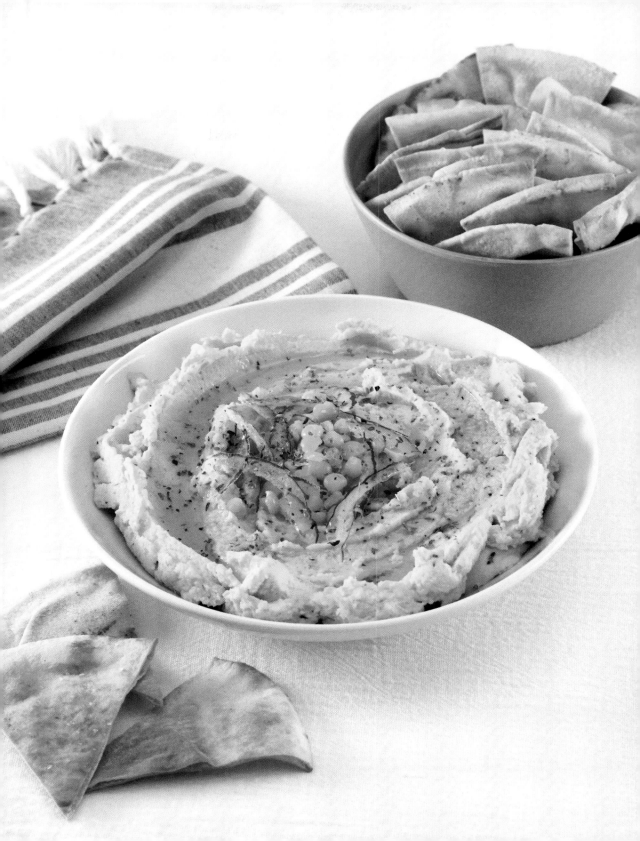

Layered Baked Feta and Tomato

This dish, also called bouyiourdi, is a hot, cheesy Greek fondue that's perfect with crusty bread. It's simple to put together, but the rich flavors taste like you spent all day in the kitchen. If you don't have a banana pepper, you can use a yellow bell pepper in its place.

SERVES 4

1 large tomato, diced, divided

$\frac{1}{2}$ cup grated kasseri or Gouda cheese, divided

$\frac{1}{2}$ cup crumbled feta cheese

1 small banana pepper, seeded and sliced into $\frac{1}{4}$" slices

1 tablespoon extra-virgin olive oil

$\frac{1}{4}$ teaspoon crushed red pepper

$\frac{1}{2}$ teaspoon dried oregano

1. Preheat oven to 400°F. Place one-half of tomatoes in a medium ramekin. Top tomatoes with ¼ cup kasseri and then feta. Top cheeses with remaining one-half tomatoes. Top tomatoes with remaining ¼ cup kasseri and peppers.

2. Drizzle oil over peppers and sprinkle with crushed red pepper and oregano.

3. Cover the ramekin tightly with foil and bake for 20 minutes or until the cheese is bubbling. Serve immediately.

Calories 182

PER SERVING

Fat 14g
Sodium 415mg
Carbohydrates 4.5g
Fiber 1g
Sugar 3g
Protein 10g

Eggplant Caponata

Serve this tasty dish on small slices of Italian bread as an appetizer or use as a filling in sandwiches or wraps. The pine nuts are a tasty and nutritious part of the recipe—they provide iron, magnesium, and antioxidants. Making this in a slow cooker means that you can put it together and then let it cook while you prepare other things.

SERVES 12

2 medium eggplants

1 teaspoon olive oil

1 medium red onion, peeled and diced

4 cloves garlic, peeled and minced

1 stalk celery, ends trimmed and diced

2 medium tomatoes, diced

2 tablespoons nonpareil capers

2 tablespoons pine nuts, toasted

1 teaspoon crushed red pepper

1/4 cup red wine vinegar

1. Pierce eggplants with a fork. Cover and cook 2 hours on high in a 4- to 5-quart slow cooker.

2. Allow eggplants to cool. Peel off skin, slice each in half, and remove seeds. Discard skin and seeds.

3. Process eggplant in a food processor until smooth. Set aside.

4. Heat oil in a large skillet over medium-high heat. Sauté onion, garlic, and celery until onion is soft, about 5–7 minutes. Add eggplant and tomatoes. Sauté for 3 minutes.

5. Return to slow cooker and add capers, pine nuts, crushed red pepper, and vinegar. Stir to combine. Cover and cook on low 30 minutes. Stir prior to serving.

Calories 45

PER SERVING

Fat 1.5g
Sodium 60mg
Carbohydrates 7g
Fiber 3g
Sugar 3g
Protein 1g

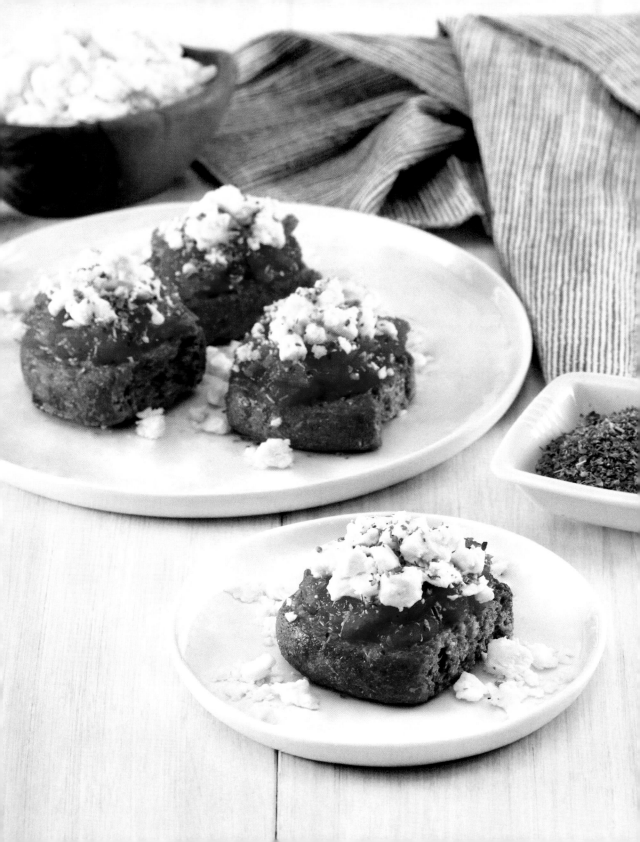

Greek Bruschetta

Dakos, or rusks, are hard twice-baked slices of bread. You can find rusks at Greek or Middle Eastern grocers. Try to use the highest quality ingredients you can find so they can shine in this simple dish.

SERVES 4

4 medium rusks

1 clove garlic, peeled

3 tablespoons extra-virgin olive oil

1 large tomato, peeled and grated

1/4 cup crumbled feta cheese

1 teaspoon dried oregano

1　Sprinkle some water over each rusk to soften them slightly. Then firmly rub the garlic clove over each rusk to infuse garlic flavor.

2　Drizzle oil evenly over rusks and let them absorb the oil for 4–5 minutes.

3　Top rusks with tomato, feta, and a sprinkle of oregano. Serve at room temperature.

Calories 170

PER SERVING

Fat 13g
Sodium 115mg
Carbohydrates 10g
Fiber 1g
Sugar 2g
Protein 3g

Stuffed Grape Leaves

Stuffed grape leaves, also called dolmades, are a Greek and Turkish dish that consists of savory rice stuffed into grape leaves and baked in a sauce. Grape leaves are low in calories but high in fiber, making them a great choice when you're trying to manage weight.

SERVES 12

1/4 cup plus 2 tablespoons extra-virgin olive oil, divided

1 medium onion, peeled and chopped

1 cup long-grain rice

1 teaspoon tomato paste, diluted in 1/2 cup warm water

1/2 cup chopped fresh parsley

1/2 cup chopped fresh dill

1/4 cup chopped fresh mint

1/3 cup pine nuts

1 tablespoon fresh lemon juice

2 1/2 teaspoons salt

3/4 teaspoon freshly ground black pepper

40 medium jarred grape leaves, rinsed and stemmed

1 1/2 cups vegetable stock, heated

2 medium lemons, thinly sliced

1 Heat 2 tablespoons oil in a large skillet over medium-low heat for 30 seconds. Add onion and cook for 5–7 minutes or until translucent. Stir in rice and cook for 3 minutes. Stir in tomato paste. Cook for 3–4 minutes more or until most of the liquid has been absorbed by the rice. Take the skillet off heat, stir in parsley, dill, mint, pine nuts, and lemon juice. Season with salt and pepper and allow the rice mixture to cool.

2 Preheat oven to 325°F. Place a grape leaf on a work surface with seam-side up. Place 1 teaspoon of the rice mixture in the middle bottom part of the leaf. Fold the bottom of leaf over the filling, and then tuck in the sides of leaf. Roll leaf into a cigar shape. Repeat with remaining leaves. Place stuffed leaves snugly into an ungreased medium roasting pan with a lid.

3 Pour remaining 1/4 cup oil and stock over stuffed leaves. Top with a layer of lemon slices. Cover the pan and bake for 30–35 minutes. Remove lemon slices before serving. Serve at room temperature.

Calories 160

PER SERVING

Fat 10g
Sodium 500mg
Carbohydrates 16g
Fiber 2g
Sugar 2g
Protein 2g

FINDING GRAPE LEAVES

If you don't have access to fresh grape leaves, there are many jarred options available in Greek or Middle Eastern grocery stores. Remember to rinse the jarred grape leaves before using them.

Roasted Peppers, Eggplant, and Tomato Dip

This dip is sometimes called taltsenes, *which is a Greek word that refers to pounding or mashing with a mortar and pestle. This richly flavored dish should be served with crusty breads and salty cheeses. The eggplant provides antioxidants and a wide range of vitamins and minerals.*

SERVES 6

1 medium tomato

2 medium Italian eggplants or 4 long Japanese eggplants

2 medium red shepherd peppers

2 teaspoons salt, divided

3 cloves garlic, peeled and minced

1 teaspoon red wine vinegar

¾ cup extra-virgin olive oil

1. Preheat a gas or charcoal grill to medium-high heat. Wrap tomato in foil. Pierce skins of eggplants a few times with a knife. Place eggplants, peppers, and tomato on grill. Cook the eggplants for 20–30 minutes or until skin is completely charred and inside is soft. Grill peppers until charred on all sides. Grill tomato in foil for 20 minutes.

2. Place charred peppers in a medium bowl and cover tightly with plastic wrap. Allow peppers to cool for 15 minutes. Using your hands, remove and discard charred skins. Slit peppers in half; remove and discard seeds and stem. Chop peppers.

3. Let eggplants cool for 10 minutes. Cut open each eggplant lengthwise and scoop out softened flesh, discarding charred skin. Peel and discard skin off tomato and chop the flesh.

4. In a mortar, add ½ teaspoon salt and garlic. Pound garlic into a mash with the pestle. Using the pestle, blend in eggplant flesh and vinegar. Blend in peppers and tomato. The mixture should not be completely smooth.

5. Stir oil in slowly and continue to blend until well incorporated. Season dip with remaining 1½ teaspoons salt and serve at room temperature.

Calories 340

PER SERVING

Fat 28g
Sodium 780mg
Carbohydrates 18g
Fiber 7g
Sugar 11g
Protein 4g

MORTAR AND PESTLE

A mortar and pestle is a worthwhile investment for your kitchen. It can be used to mix an array of dips and dressings and grind spices and nuts.

Parsley Spread

This unusual spread is a refreshing change of pace from heavy cream-based options. Grab a bunch of fresh parsley from your local farmers' market, grocery store—or maybe even your own herb garden! Serve this spread on crostini, pita chips, or fresh vegetable sticks.

SERVES 8

4 slices stale bread, crusts removed

2 cups chopped fresh parsley

3 scallions, ends trimmed and chopped

1/2 cup extra-virgin olive oil

1/4 cup fresh lemon juice

1 tablespoon white wine vinegar

1 teaspoon dried oregano

1 teaspoon salt

1/2 teaspoon freshly ground black pepper

1. In a medium bowl, moisten bread with a little water. Squeeze to drain excess water.

2. Process parsley and scallions in a food processor. Slowly add bread, oil, lemon juice, vinegar, oregano, salt, and pepper. Continue processing until smooth. Refrigerate or serve at room temperature.

Calories 180

PER SERVING

Fat 15g
Sodium 380mg
Carbohydrates 10g
Fiber 1g
Sugar 1g
Protein 2g

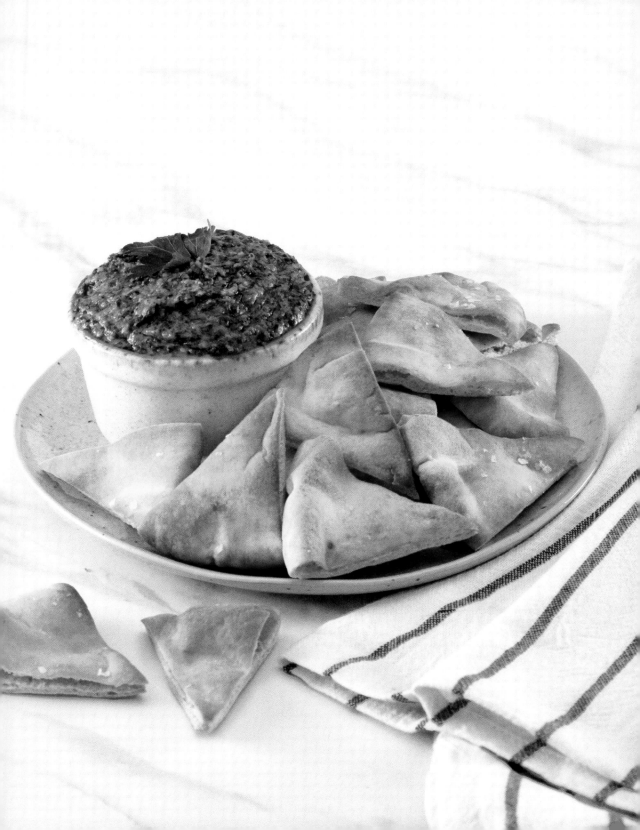

Phyllo-Wrapped Shrimp

Frozen store-bought appetizers never quite capture the flavors of a freshly made one. Working with phyllo dough doesn't have to be difficult—try this simple recipe to become more familiar with it. Serve this dish with a spicy cocktail sauce.

SERVES 4

12 medium fresh shrimp, shelled (tails on) and deveined

2 tablespoons extra-virgin olive oil

1/2 teaspoon salt

1/2 teaspoon freshly ground black pepper

2 cloves garlic, peeled and minced

1/2 teaspoon sweet paprika

2 cups sunflower oil for frying

4 sheets phyllo pastry

1 teaspoon cornstarch, dissolved in 1 teaspoon room temperature water

1 Slit the inside curve of each shrimp 3 or 4 times to straighten it out. In a medium bowl, combine the olive oil, salt, pepper, garlic, and paprika. Toss shrimp in mixture. Set aside.

2 In a deep skillet over medium-high heat, bring 2 inches of sunflower oil to 360°F. Adjust heat to keep temperature at 360°F while frying.

3 Cut phyllo sheets into 6" × 4" × 4" triangles and lay them out on a work surface. Work quickly because you don't want the phyllo to dry out. Place a shrimp near the left corner of the phyllo with tail exposed and body lying inside the phyllo. Fold the phyllo over shrimp and tuck it tightly under the top of shrimp. Fold the top part of the phyllo over to cover shrimp. Finally, roll up the phyllo until the roll is complete. Dab your finger into cornstarch paste and seal the end of the phyllo. Repeat with remaining shrimp.

4 Fry shrimp rolls in batches for 3 minutes or until golden, and shrimp is cooked through. Place shrimp on a tray lined with paper towels to absorb excess oil. Serve immediately.

Calories 180

PER SERVING

Fat 13g
Sodium 480mg
Carbohydrates 12g
Fiber 0g
Sugar 0g
Protein 4g

Zucchini Patties

The Greek word for this dish is kolokithokeftedes. *These baked zucchini fritters are great with a side of your favorite feta or yogurt dip or sauce. Zucchini is naturally low in calories and provides fiber to aid in digestion.*

SERVES 6

3 medium zucchini, trimmed and grated

1 teaspoon salt

6 tablespoons extra-virgin olive oil, divided

6 scallions, ends trimmed and finely chopped

1 clove garlic, peeled and minced

1 large egg, beaten

2 tablespoons chopped fresh mint

1 tablespoon chopped fresh dill

1 tablespoon chopped fresh parsley

$1/2$ cup bread crumbs

$1/4$ cup grated graviera or Gruyère cheese

$1/2$ cup crumbled feta cheese

$1/2$ teaspoon freshly ground black pepper

1 tablespoon baking powder

1. Put zucchini and salt into a colander. Cover the colander with plastic wrap and place over a bowl to catch the drained water. Refrigerate zucchini for at least 3 hours. Squeeze any remaining liquid from zucchini with your hands or wring out in a clean tea towel. Try to get zucchini as dry as possible.

2. Preheat oven to 425°F. Heat 3 tablespoons oil in a medium skillet over medium heat for 30 seconds. Add scallions and garlic and cook for 5–7 minutes. Take skillet off heat and allow scallion mixture to cool.

3. In a large bowl, combine cooled scallion mixture, egg, mint, dill, parsley, bread crumbs, graviera, feta, pepper, and baking powder. If mixture is too wet, add a few more bread crumbs. If mixture is too dry, add a little more oil.

4. Using your hands, form mixture into small patties, each about 3" wide. You should have enough for twelve to fourteen patties. Place patties on a greased baking sheet and brush tops with remaining 3 tablespoons oil.

5. Bake for 8–10 minutes on the middle rack. Flip patties over and bake for 8–10 minutes more or until golden. Serve warm or at room temperature.

Calories 250

PER SERVING

Fat 20g
Sodium 620mg
Carbohydrates 12g
Fiber 1g
Sugar 3g
Protein 7g

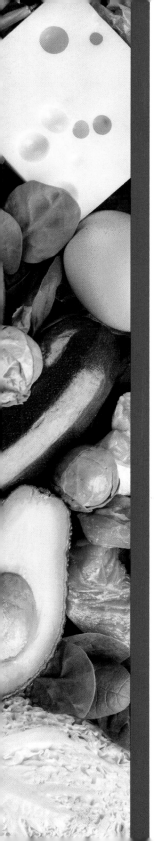

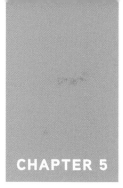

CHAPTER 5

Side Dishes

While the main dish is the star of a meal, side dishes can provide important variety in flavors, colors, and textures to complement it. Opt for a simple Amaranth Greens salad, slow-cooked Braised Lentils, or Sautéed Mushrooms to go alongside whatever else you're making. Try to balance rich and light flavors, and think about how the foods will look together when plated. While some side dishes can pile on the calories, the options in this chapter will help you meet your daily goals while also providing countless nutritional benefits.

Amaranth Greens

These beautiful red, purple, and green leaves will brighten any dinner table. The name amaranth *comes from the Greek word* amárantos, *meaning "the never-fading," because the flowers of this plant stay colorful even after harvest. And best of all, they contain a lot of vitamin C and iron. If you can't find amaranth greens, use dandelion greens.*

SERVES 4

3 teaspoons salt, divided	3 cups amaranth greens, roughly chopped	½ cup extra-virgin olive oil 1 tablespoon fresh lemon juice

1 Fill a large pot two-thirds with water and set over medium-high heat. Bring water to a boil and add 2 teaspoons of salt and the amaranth. Reduce heat to medium and cook for 10–12 minutes or until the amaranth stems are fork-tender. Drain amaranth and discard cooking water.

2 In a medium bowl, combine amaranth, oil, and lemon juice. Season with the remaining 1 teaspoon salt, and serve warm.

Calories 240

PER SERVING

Fat 25g
Sodium 602mg
Carbohydrates 2.5g
Fiber 3g
Sugar 0.5g
Protein 1g

WHAT ARE AMARANTH GREENS?

Amaranth greens, which grow wild in the Mediterranean region, are loaded with iron and are good for your blood. Look for amaranth at Asian markets. Young amaranth greens can be eaten raw, but mature greens need to be cooked because they are bitter.

Sautéed Artichoke Hearts

Artichokes are low in calories so they are a great side dish for keeping your daily calorie counts on track. Marjoram tastes a little sweeter than thyme, and makes this savory dish really mouthwatering. Fresh baby artichokes cut in half work well for this recipe.

SERVES 6

½ cup all-purpose flour

½ cup skim milk

3 cups artichoke hearts, cut in half

1 tablespoon chopped fresh marjoram

2 tablespoons chopped fresh rosemary leaves

2 tablespoons olive oil

1 Place flour in a medium shallow dish and milk in another medium shallow dish. Dip artichoke hearts in flour, then in milk, then in flour again. Place coated artichoke hearts on a rack. Sprinkle with marjoram and rosemary.

2 Heat oil in a large skillet over medium heat. Sauté artichokes on all sides until golden brown, about 10 minutes. Drain on rack covered with paper towels before serving.

Calories 110

PER SERVING

Fat 4.5g
Sodium 310mg
Carbohydrates 13g
Fiber 1g
Sugar 3g
Protein 4g

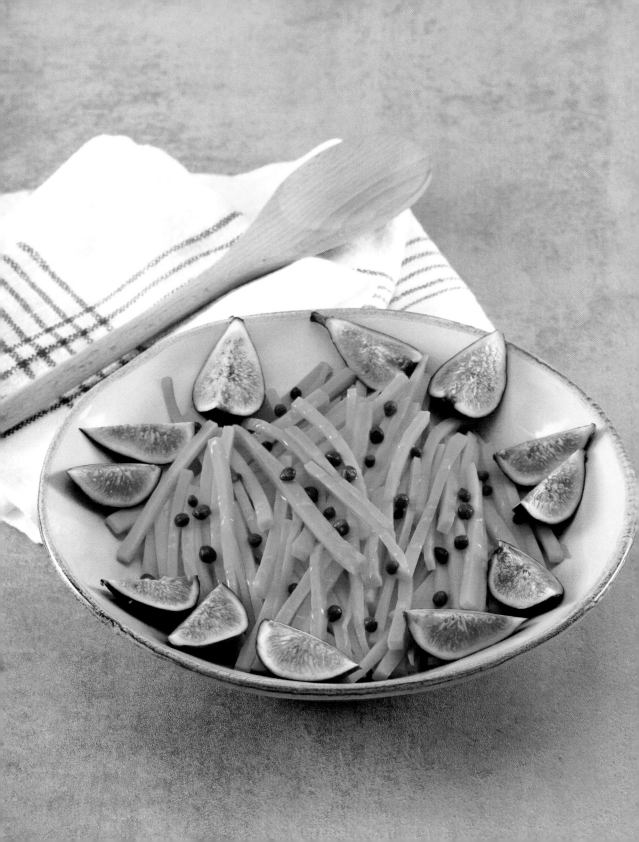

Citrus-Steamed Carrots

Figs and carrots go together surprisingly well. The citrus and capers provide a tart contrast to the sweetness. Plus, you're getting a wealth of key vitamins and minerals and other nutrients from carrots, such as beta carotene, vitamin K1, fiber, and potassium.

SERVES 6

1 cup orange juice

2 tablespoons fresh lemon juice

2 tablespoons fresh lime juice

1 pound carrots, peeled and julienned

3 large figs, cut into wedges

1 tablespoon extra-virgin olive oil

1 tablespoon capers

1 In a large saucepan, combine orange, lemon, and lime juices over medium-high heat. Add carrots, cover, and steam until al dente, about 6 minutes. Remove from heat and cool.

2 Transfer carrots to a serving platter and arrange figs around carrots. Sprinkle oil and capers on top and serve.

Calories 100

PER SERVING

Fat 2.5g
Sodium 85mg
Carbohydrates 18g
Fiber 3g
Sugar 13g
Protein 1g

Grilled Asparagus with Roasted Peppers and Feta

Asparagus has a distinct flavor that can complement a lot of main dishes. It is another vegetable that's rich in fiber, plus also contains folate and vitamins K, A, and C. Keep an eye on the asparagus while grilling because they burn easily. For instructions on how to prepare your own roasted red peppers, see the sidebar with Chickpea Salad with Roasted Red Peppers and Green Beans in Chapter 10.

SERVES 4

½ pound asparagus, woody ends trimmed

4 tablespoons extra-virgin olive oil, divided

½ teaspoon salt

¼ teaspoon freshly ground black pepper

3 tablespoons vegetable oil

1 roasted red pepper, chopped

½ cup crumbled feta cheese

1 In a large bowl, combine asparagus, 2 tablespoons olive oil, salt, and pepper. Toss to coat asparagus.

2 Preheat a gas or charcoal grill to medium-high heat. When grill is ready, dip a clean tea towel in vegetable oil and wipe the grill's surface.

3 Grill asparagus for 2 minutes per side. Arrange on a serving platter and top with roasted red pepper. Sprinkle cheese on top and drizzle with remaining 2 tablespoons olive oil. Serve immediately.

Calories 280

PER SERVING

Fat 29g
Sodium 570mg
Carbohydrates 4g
Fiber 1g
Sugar 3g
Protein 4g

Broiled Eggplant

It's likely that you have had eggplant Parmesan on more than one occasion, but there are lots of other ways to prepare the vegetable. This dish highlights eggplant's mild flavor while keeping the calorie count low. One prep note: If you use small Chinese eggplants, cut them in half rather than into slices.

SERVES 6

4 small eggplants, sliced lengthwise into 1/8" pieces

4 cloves garlic, peeled and minced

1 tablespoon olive oil

3/4 teaspoon salt, divided

1/2 teaspoon freshly ground black pepper

1. Preheat broiler.

2. In a large bowl, toss eggplant with garlic, oil, 1/2 teaspoon salt, and pepper. Place eggplant on a broiler pan or baking sheet.

3. Broil 5 minutes per side until golden brown outside and soft inside. Season with remaining 1/4 teaspoon salt. Serve immediately.

Calories 110

PER SERVING

Fat 3g
Sodium 300mg
Carbohydrates 22g
Fiber 10g
Sugar 12g
Protein 4g

Lemon Garlic Green Beans

Green beans are tasty prepared a lot of different ways—raw, blanched, cooked in a casserole, and so on. This recipe slow-cooks them and brightens the flavors with lemon zest and sliced garlic.

SERVES 4

1½ pounds green beans, trimmed

3 tablespoons olive oil

3 large shallots, peeled and cut into thin wedges

6 cloves garlic, peeled and sliced

1 tablespoon grated lemon zest

½ teaspoon salt

½ teaspoon freshly ground black pepper

½ cup water

Spray a 4- to 5-quart slow cooker with nonstick cooking spray. Place green beans in slow cooker. Add remaining ingredients over beans. Cover and cook on high 4–6 hours or on low 8–10 hours. Serve warm.

Calories 160

PER SERVING

Fat 11g
Sodium 310mg
Carbohydrates 17g
Fiber 6g
Sugar 7g
Protein 4g

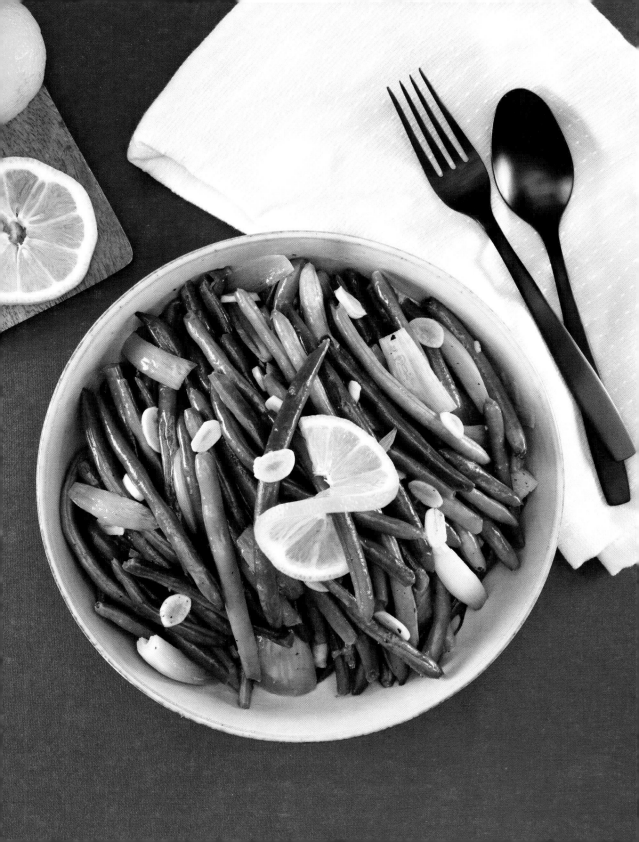

Wax Beans with Roasted Garlic, Capers, and Parsley

Pale yellow wax beans have a mild flavor that can absorb the other, bolder flavors in this dish. If you can't find wax beans, green beans (or a combination of green and yellow beans) also work in this recipe.

SERVES 6

1 pound wax beans, trimmed

2½ teaspoons salt, divided

1 cup fresh parsley leaves

3 tablespoons capers, rinsed

1½ teaspoons grated lemon zest

1 teaspoon Dijon mustard

⅓ cup extra-virgin olive oil

1 whole head garlic, roasted and cloves extracted (see sidebar)

1 teaspoon dried oregano

1½ teaspoons red wine vinegar

½ teaspoon freshly ground black pepper

1. Fill a large pot two-thirds with water and bring to a boil over medium-high heat. Add beans and 1½ teaspoons of salt. Bring water back to a boil, and then reduce heat to medium. Cook beans for 6–7 minutes or until they are cooked, but not soft. Remove beans from water and place them in an ice bath to stop the cooking process. When beans are cool, remove them from the ice bath and set aside.

2. In a food processor, combine parsley, capers, lemon zest, mustard, and oil. Process ingredients to make the dressing.

3. In a large bowl, combine beans, garlic, oregano, vinegar, and dressing. Toss beans to coat them, and then season with remaining 1 teaspoon salt and pepper. Serve warm.

Calories 150

PER SERVING

Fat 13g
Sodium 700mg
Carbohydrates 7g
Fiber 3g
Sugar 3g
Protein 2g

HOW TO ROAST GARLIC

Roasting your own garlic is easy. Preheat the oven to 350°F. Cut the top off a whole head of garlic, removing just enough to expose the cloves inside. Place the garlic on a sheet of aluminum foil and lightly drizzle it with olive oil and then add a sprinkle of salt. Wrap the foil around the garlic and roast for 35–50 minutes. Allow the garlic to cool. Remove each clove with a knife, or squeeze the whole head until the cloves pop out.

Braised Lentils

Lentils aren't just for soup! Try this fiber-packed side dish for a hearty option alongside a protein. Always wait to salt lentils until the end of cooking because salt can make them tough.

SERVES 6

1/4 cup extra-virgin olive oil

1/4 cup finely chopped red onion

1/2 cup finely chopped celery

1/2 cup finely chopped peeled carrots

1 1/2 cups dried green or brown lentils, rinsed

1 bay leaf

2 sprigs fresh oregano

2 sprigs fresh parsley

4 cups vegetable stock

1 1/2 teaspoons salt

1/2 teaspoon freshly ground black pepper

1 Heat oil in a medium pot over medium-high heat for 30 seconds. Add red onion, celery, and carrots. Cook for 2–3 minutes until vegetables soften. Add lentils, bay leaf, oregano, parsley, and stock. Cover pot, and reduce heat to medium-low. Cook for 30–40 minutes or until almost all the liquid is absorbed.

2 Discard bay leaf, oregano, and parsley, and season lentils with salt and pepper. Serve warm.

Calories 260

PER SERVING

Fat 10g
Sodium 660mg
Carbohydrates 31g
Fiber 8g
Sugar 2g
Protein 13g

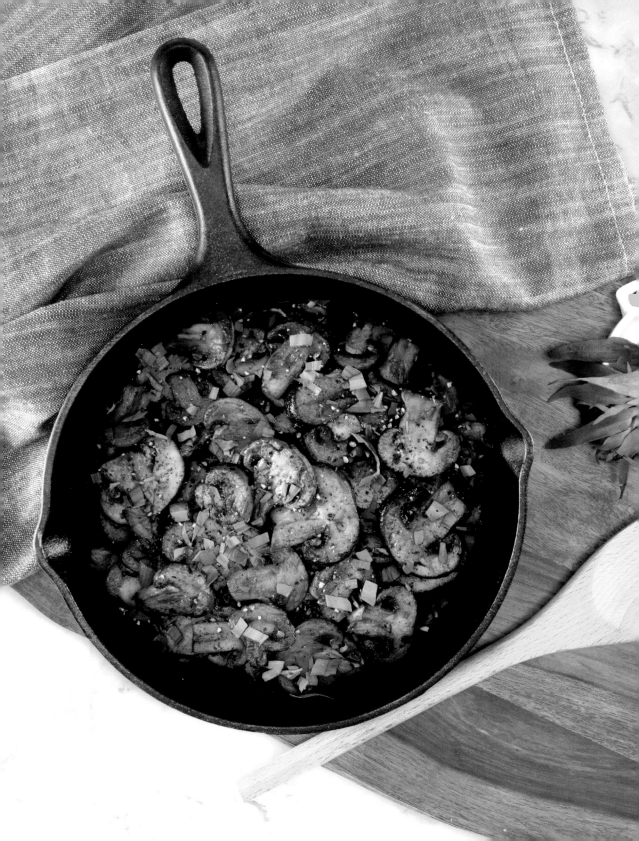

Sautéed Mushrooms

This quick and easy side dish is perfect for a busy weeknight. In addition to a lovely earthy flavor, you'll also enjoy the B vitamins that mushrooms provide. A good assortment of mushrooms to try in this recipe includes button, oyster, enoki, shiitake, and portobello.

SERVES 6

1 tablespoon olive oil

1½ pounds assorted mushrooms, sliced

1 medium shallot, peeled and diced

4 cloves garlic, peeled and minced

¼ cup dry white wine

1 teaspoon freshly ground black pepper

1 teaspoon tarragon leaves

1 Heat oil in a large skillet over medium heat, then add mushrooms, shallot, and garlic. Sauté about 10 minutes.

2 Add wine to pan and cook for 10 minutes more, until reduced by half. Remove from heat and sprinkle with pepper and tarragon before serving.

Calories 60

PER SERVING

Fat 2.5g
Sodium 10mg
Carbohydrates 7g
Fiber 1g
Sugar 2g
Protein 3g

Asparagus Gratin

Asparagus tastes best when it's consumed in season. Remember to trim or peel the woody ends; they are fibrous and most people would rather not eat them. If you can find it, use Metsovone cheese instead of Gouda. It's a semi-hard smoked cheese made with cow's milk in Greece.

SERVES 6

1 teaspoon salt, divided

2 pounds asparagus, woody ends trimmed

2 tablespoons unsalted butter, divided

2 tablespoons all-purpose flour

1½ cups warm whole milk

½ cup grated Gouda cheese

¼ cup grated Romano cheese

½ teaspoon freshly ground black pepper

½ cup bread crumbs

1. Preheat oven to 375°F. Fill a large pot two-thirds with water and set over medium-high heat. Bring water to a boil and add ½ teaspoon salt and asparagus. Return water to a boil and cook asparagus for 2 minutes. Remove asparagus from water and place it in an ice bath to stop the cooking process. Remove asparagus from ice bath when cooled and set aside.

2. Melt 1 tablespoon of butter in a medium skillet over medium heat. Stir in flour and cook for 2 minutes. Add milk and keep stirring until the sauce thickens to a creamy texture. Take sauce off heat and stir in cheeses. Season with remaining ½ teaspoon salt and pepper and keep warm.

3. Grease a large baking dish with remaining 1 tablespoon butter. Lay asparagus lengthwise in the dish with half of the tips pointing in one direction and the other half pointing in the opposite direction. Pour sauce over asparagus, leaving the tips of spears exposed. Sprinkle bread crumbs over sauce. Bake asparagus for 30 minutes or until the top is golden brown. Serve hot.

Calories 200

PER SERVING

Fat 10g
Sodium 630mg
Carbohydrates 17g
Fiber 3g
Sugar 6g
Protein 11g

ASPARAGUS IN ANCIENT TIMES

Asparagus is derived from the Greek word meaning "sprout" and has grown in the Mediterranean region since antiquity. It was used for medicinal purposes and as an aphrodisiac.

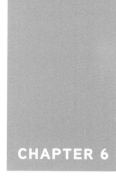

CHAPTER 6

Chicken and Poultry Main Dishes

Protein-rich, low in calories, and flavorful: Chicken and poultry dishes fit well in the Mediterranean diet for many reasons. The recipes in this chapter call on fresh herbs and spices to create delicious, savory main dishes that work well for a family on a weeknight or dinner guests on a weekend. You'll find the dishes easy to make but satisfying and filling—plus, they won't take your diet off track. The recipes range from the more traditional (Tuscan Chicken and White Beans) to the unique (Chicken with Figs).

Chicken Skewers

These Chicken Skewers are traditionally served with lightly grilled pita bread and tzatziki. To round out the meal, you can add vegetable chunks to the skewers as well.

SERVES 8

2 pounds boneless, skinless chicken thighs, cut into 1" cubes

1/3 cup extra-virgin olive oil

2 medium onions, peeled and grated

4 cloves garlic, peeled and minced

2 tablespoons grated lemon zest

1 teaspoon dried oregano

1 teaspoon chopped fresh rosemary leaves

1 teaspoon salt

1 teaspoon freshly ground black pepper

2 tablespoons fresh lemon juice

1. In a large bowl, combine chicken, olive oil, onions, garlic, lemon zest, oregano, rosemary, salt, and pepper. Toss to coat. Cover bowl with plastic wrap and refrigerate 8 hours or overnight. Take chicken out of the refrigerator 30 minutes before skewering.

2. Preheat a gas or charcoal grill to medium-high heat. When grill is ready, dip a clean tea towel in vegetable oil and wipe the grill's surface.

3. Put chicken onto wooden or metal skewers; each skewer should hold four pieces.

4. Place skewers on grill and cook for 3–4 minutes per side or until chicken is no longer pink inside.

5. Drizzle lemon juice over skewers and serve.

Calories 140

PER SERVING

Fat 5g
Sodium 390mg
Carbohydrates 1g
Fiber 0g
Sugar 0g
Protein 23g

Chicken Galantine

Galantine is often a French specialty dish of stuffed meat. To change up this version, you can encase the ground chicken mixture in roasted eggplant instead of using skin. This will add additional flavor to the chicken.

SERVES 6

1 small whole chicken

1/2 pound ground chicken

1 large egg white

1/4 cup chopped pistachios

8 dates, chopped

1 shallot, peeled and minced

2 cloves garlic, peeled and minced

1 teaspoon dried oregano

1 teaspoon dried marjoram

1/8 teaspoon freshly ground black pepper

1/8 teaspoon kosher salt

1. Preheat oven to 325°F. Carefully remove all the skin from the whole chicken by making a slit down the back and loosening the skin with your fingers (keep the skin intact as much as possible); set chicken and skin aside. Remove the breast from bone.

2. Mix the ground chicken, egg white, nuts, dates, shallot, garlic, oregano, marjoram, pepper, and salt together.

3. Lay out the skin, then lay the breast lengthwise at the center. Spoon ground chicken mixture on top, and fold over the rest of skin. Lightly spray a loaf pan with nonstick cooking spray. Gently place loaf in pan and bake for 1 1/2–2 hours until the internal temperature reaches 170°F. Let cool, then slice and serve.

Calories 240

PER SERVING

Fat 8g
Sodium 170mg
Carbohydrates 10g
Fiber 1g
Sugar 8g
Protein 32g

Pomegranate-Glazed Chicken

Seasoning chicken with pomegranate not only tastes great—it provides a healthy dose of antioxidants. Make sure you use pure pomegranate juice in this recipe because other versions can contain a lot of added sugar and calories. Mastiha is a spice that can be found at Greek or Middle Eastern grocery stores.

SERVES 4

4 (6-ounce) bone-in, skinless chicken breasts

½ teaspoon salt

½ teaspoon freshly ground black pepper

2 cups pomegranate juice

⅛ teaspoon ground mastiha

2 teaspoons grated orange zest

3 cloves garlic, peeled and smashed

1 teaspoon dried rosemary

1 Preheat oven to 375°F. Season chicken with salt and pepper and place on a baking sheet lined with parchment paper. Bake chicken for 25–30 minutes or until the internal temperature reaches 180°F.

2 In a small pan over medium-high heat, combine pomegranate juice, mastiha, orange zest, garlic, and rosemary. Bring mixture to a boil, reduce heat to medium-low, and cook until sauce reduces to ¼ cup and has a syruplike consistency. Remove garlic and take sauce off heat.

3 Brush chicken with sauce before serving.

Calories 240

PER SERVING

Fat 3.5g
Sodium 370mg
Carbohydrates 19g
Fiber 0g
Sugar 17g
Protein 31g

MAKE YOUR OWN FRESH POMEGRANATE JUICE

You can easily make your own pomegranate juice. Slice 3 or 4 pomegranates in half. With the seed side over a bowl, tap each pomegranate bottom with a wooden spoon to release the seeds. You'll need to tap several times to release all the seeds. Remove any white pith from the bowl. Put the seeds in a food processor and process for 5 minutes. Strain the juice with a fine mesh sieve to remove the pits.

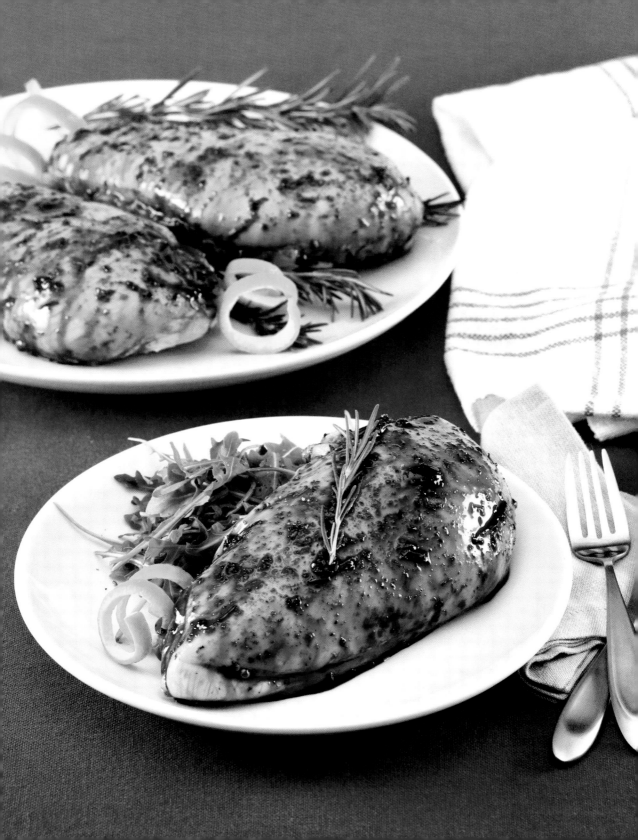

Chicken with Figs

Figs are rich in a variety of minerals, including potassium, calcium, magnesium, copper, and iron. They offer a mild sweetness that pairs well with sweet potatoes and garlic. This recipe was inspired by the traditional Moroccan tagine.

SERVES 8

- 1/2 pound boneless, skinless chicken thighs, cubed
- 3/4 pound boneless, skinless chicken breasts, cubed
- 3/4 cup dried figs
- 1 medium sweet potato, peeled and diced
- 1 medium onion, peeled and chopped
- 3 cloves garlic, peeled and minced
- 2 teaspoons ground cumin
- 1 teaspoon coriander
- 1/2 teaspoon cayenne pepper
- 1/2 teaspoon ground ginger
- 1/2 teaspoon turmeric
- 1/2 teaspoon ground orange peel
- 1/2 teaspoon freshly ground black pepper
- 2 3/4 cups low-sodium chicken broth
- 1/4 cup orange juice

1. Sauté chicken in a large dry nonstick skillet over medium-high heat until it starts to turn white, about 3 minutes, and then drain.

2. Place chicken and remaining ingredients into an ungreased 4- to 5-quart slow cooker and stir to combine. Cover and cook on low 6 hours. Stir again before serving.

Calories 150

PER SERVING

Fat 2.5g
Sodium 75mg
Carbohydrates 15g
Fiber 2g
Sugar 9g
Protein 17g

Balsamic Chicken and Spinach

Balsamic vinegar is delicious in any dish, but is especially well paired with chicken. This simple slow cooker recipe is flavorful and filling but contains only 130 calories per serving! Serve this tangy and nutritious dish with rice pilaf.

SERVES 4

3/4 pound boneless, skinless chicken breasts, cut into strips

1/4 cup balsamic vinegar

4 cloves garlic, peeled and minced

1 tablespoon minced fresh oregano

1 tablespoon minced fresh parsley

1/2 teaspoon freshly ground black pepper

5 ounces baby spinach

1 Place chicken, vinegar, garlic, oregano, parsley, and pepper into a 4- to 5-quart slow cooker. Stir to combine. Cover and cook on low 6 hours.

2 Add baby spinach and cover again. Cook until spinach is wilted, about 15 minutes. Stir before serving.

Calories 130

PER SERVING

Fat 2.5g
Sodium 70mg
Carbohydrates 5g
Fiber 1g
Sugar 2g
Protein 20g

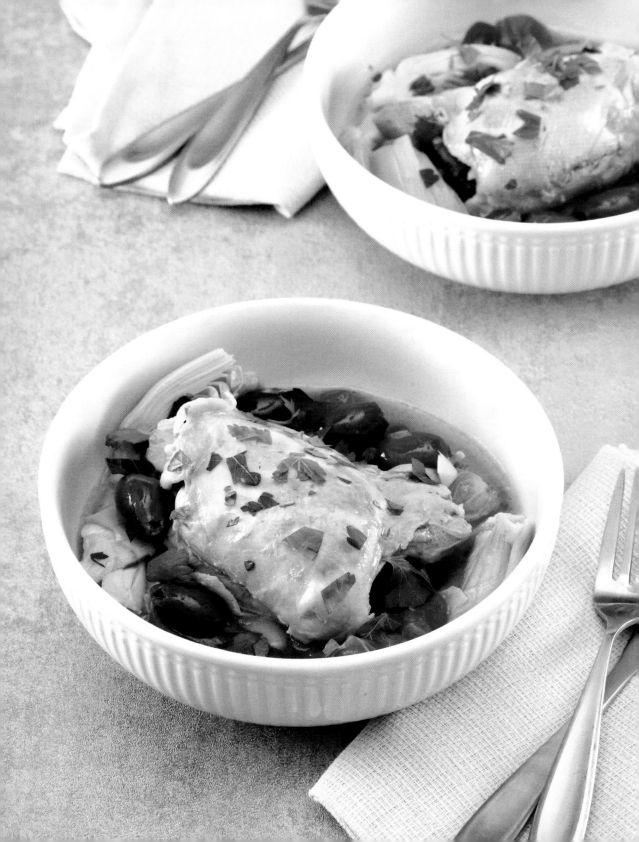

Five-Ingredient Greek Chicken

If you've got these five ingredients in your kitchen, you've got a gorgeously slow-cooked meal waiting to feed you and your family—at only 180 calories a serving! This is the perfect meal to serve with crusty French bread on a cold, rainy night.

SERVES 6

6 (5-ounce) bone-in, skinless chicken thighs

$\frac{1}{2}$ cup pitted Kalamata olives

1 (6.5-ounce) jar artichoke hearts in olive oil, undrained

1 pint cherry tomatoes

$\frac{1}{4}$ cup chopped fresh parsley

1. Place chicken, olives, artichokes and artichoke oil, and cherry tomatoes in a 4- to 5-quart slow cooker.

2. Cover and cook on low 4–6 hours. Serve in large bowls garnished with parsley.

Calories 180

PER SERVING

Fat 8g
Sodium 410mg
Carbohydrates 7g
Fiber 2g
Sugar 1g
Protein 18g

Sage Ricotta Chicken Breasts

Fresh sage adds a distinctly bold flavor to this chicken dish. If you have difficulty spreading the cheese mixture under the skin, you can lift the chicken skin completely off, spoon on the cheese mixture, and replace the skin.

SERVES 6

½ cup part-skim ricotta cheese

6 fresh sage leaves, sliced

1 large egg white

6 (8-ounce) bone-in, chicken breasts with skin

¼ cup pitted chopped Niçoise olives

½ teaspoon freshly ground black pepper

1. Preheat oven to 375°F. In a small bowl, mix together ricotta, sage, and egg white.

2. Using your finger, make an opening in the skin of each breast and loosen the skin away from the breast.

3. Transfer ricotta mixture to a small zip-top plastic bag and snip off one corner. Squeeze ricotta mixture under chicken skin through the opening you made. Place chicken on a rack in a large baking dish. Roast for 30–45 minutes until the internal temperature of the chicken reaches 165°F and the outside is browned.

4. Transfer chicken to a serving platter. Top with olives and sprinkle with pepper.

Calories 230

PER SERVING

Fat 8g
Sodium 340mg
Carbohydrates 2g
Fiber 0g
Sugar 0g
Protein 36g

Spicy Turkey Breast with Fruit Chutney

The fruit chutney in this recipe brings a gentle and natural sweetness to this protein-packed turkey breast. Almost any type of pear will work well here, but first try either Bosc or Anjou (if available) with this recipe.

SERVES 6

2 teaspoons all-purpose flour

1/8 teaspoon freshly ground black pepper

2 medium jalapeños, seeded and minced

2 cloves garlic, peeled and minced

1 tablespoon olive oil

1 1/2 pounds whole boneless turkey breast

2 medium pears, diced

1 medium shallot, peeled and finely diced

3 tablespoons fresh lemon juice

1 tablespoon grated lemon zest

1 tablespoon honey

1. Preheat oven to 350°F. In a medium shallow dish, mix flour and black pepper together. In a blender, purée jalapeños, garlic, and oil; transfer to another medium shallow dish.

2. Spray a rack with nonstick cooking spray. Dredge turkey in flour mixture and then dip in jalapeño mixture. Place turkey on rack. Cover loosely with foil and roast for 1 hour or until cooked through. Remove foil and brown for 10 minutes.

3. For the chutney, mix pears, shallot, lemon juice, lemon zest, and honey together.

4. Thinly slice the turkey and serve with chutney.

Calories 260

PER SERVING

Fat 10g
Sodium 70mg
Carbohydrates 15g
Fiber 2g
Sugar 10g
Protein 25g

Tuscan Chicken and White Beans

Hearty white beans with warm Tuscan spices and tomatoes make this super-easy slow-cooked chicken special enough for company! Serve this traditional protein-packed dish over rice or pasta if you like.

SERVES 6

1 pound boneless, skinless chicken breasts, cut into large chunks

1 (15.5-ounce) can white beans, drained and rinsed

1 (14.5-ounce) can diced tomatoes with juice

1 (4-ounce) can mushrooms, drained

1/4 cup halved Spanish olives stuffed with pimientos

2 teaspoons onion powder

1 teaspoon garlic powder

1 teaspoon dried basil

1 teaspoon dried oregano

1 teaspoon freshly ground black pepper

1/2 teaspoon salt

2 teaspoons olive oil

1. Spray a 4- to 5-quart slow cooker with nonstick cooking spray. Add chicken, beans, tomatoes (including juice), mushrooms, olives, onion powder, garlic powder, basil, oregano, pepper, and salt. Stir to combine.

2. Drizzle oil over mixture. Cover and cook on low 6 hours or on high 3½–4 hours. Serve warm.

Calories 220

PER SERVING

Fat 4.5g
Sodium 700mg
Carbohydrates 18g
Fiber 1g
Sugar 3g
Protein 25g

THE VERSATILITY OF WHITE BEANS

White beans, which are also called navy beans, Boston beans, or Yankee beans, are small, lightly colored beans that are very mild in taste and work well in a variety of recipes. If you don't have white beans available, cannellini beans or northern beans, which are slightly larger, are excellent substitutes.

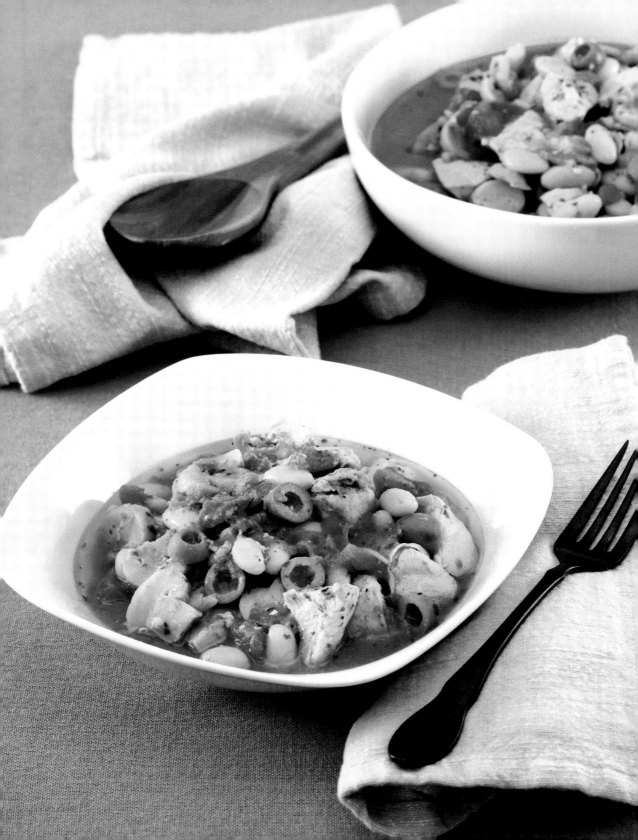

Grilled Duck Breast with Fruit Salsa

Stone fruits aren't just for pies and desserts—try them in this main dish as well. Duck breast has the best flavor when cooked rare to medium-rare. For this recipe, try using moulard duck breast if you can find it.

SERVES 6

1 tablespoon olive oil

1 teaspoon chili powder

1 1/2 pounds whole boneless duck breast

1 medium plum, diced

1 medium peach, diced

1 medium nectarine, diced

1 red onion, peeled and diced

2 teaspoons minced fresh mint

1/8 teaspoon freshly ground black pepper

1 Preheat a gas or charcoal grill to medium-high heat. Mix oil and chili powder together. Dip duck in oil mixture and cook to desired doneness on grill.

2 For the salsa, toss plums, peaches, nectarines, onion, mint, and pepper together.

3 Slice duck on the bias and serve with a spoonful of salsa.

Calories 190

PER SERVING

Fat 7g
Sodium 85mg
Carbohydrates 8g
Fiber 1g
Sugar 6g
Protein 23g

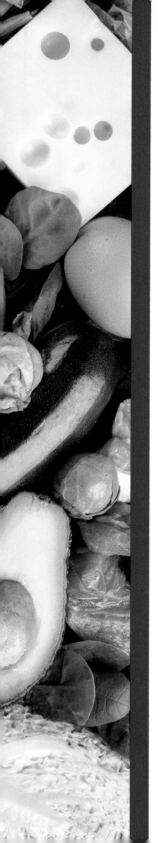

CHAPTER 7

Beef and Lamb Main Dishes

While red meat should not be eaten too often on a true Mediterranean diet, it is certainly part of the region's flavors. Lamb in particular is used in many ways. Lamb contains a lot of protein and fat, but much of the fat is composed of anti-inflammatory omega-3 fatty acids. The recipes in this chapter offer a variety of mild and bold options that remain low in calories. Try the hearty Short Ribs of Beef with Red Wine or the lighter Ginger Tomato Lamb as part of your dinner rotation.

Greek-Style Flank Steak

The garlic and scallions in this recipe impart strong flavors, especially when paired with the fresh herbs. The steak turns out juicy and packed with savory aromas and tastes.

SERVES 8

1/4 cup extra-virgin olive oil

8 cloves garlic, peeled and smashed

4 scallions, ends trimmed and chopped

1 tablespoon Dijon mustard

1/3 cup balsamic vinegar

2 bay leaves

2 tablespoons chopped fresh thyme leaves

2 tablespoons chopped fresh rosemary leaves

1 teaspoon dried oregano

1 teaspoon salt, divided

3/4 teaspoon freshly ground black pepper, divided

1 (2-pound) flank steak

1. In a food processor, process olive oil, garlic, scallions, mustard, vinegar, bay leaves, thyme, rosemary, oregano, 1/2 teaspoon salt, and 1/2 teaspoon pepper until incorporated.

2. Rub steak with marinade and place in a medium baking dish. Cover and refrigerate 3 hours. Return steak to room temperature before grilling. Wipe most of marinade off steak and season with remaining 1/2 teaspoon salt and 1/4 teaspoon pepper.

3. Preheat a gas or charcoal grill to medium-high heat. When grill is ready, dip a clean tea towel in vegetable oil and wipe the grill's surface. Grill steak for 4 minutes per side.

4. Let steak rest 5 minutes before serving.

Calories 190

PER SERVING

Fat 9g
Sodium 230mg
Carbohydrates 1g
Fiber 0g
Sugar 0g
Protein 24g

Meatballs with Mushrooms

Adding mushrooms to meatballs may seem curious, but the flavors actually pair together well. Serve these meatballs with skewers or, for a more substantial dish, provide rolls and let your guests make little meatball sandwiches.

SERVES 6

1 pound lean ground beef

1 clove garlic, peeled and minced

1/4 cup chopped celery

1/2 cup uncooked rice

1/2 cup bread crumbs

1/2 teaspoon sage

1/2 teaspoon salt

1/2 teaspoon ground white pepper

3 tablespoons vegetable oil, divided

1/2 pound mushrooms, minced

1 medium onion, peeled and minced

1 tablespoon all-purpose flour

1 cup water

1 cup tomato sauce

1. In a large bowl, combine ground beef, garlic, celery, rice, bread crumbs, sage, salt, and white pepper. Form mixture into 3/4" balls.

2. Heat 2 tablespoons vegetable oil in a large skillet over medium heat. Brown meatballs on all sides, about 1 minute per side, and place on a tray lined with paper towels to absorb excess oil.

3. Spray a 4- to 5-quart slow cooker with nonstick cooking spray. Arrange meatballs in slow cooker.

4. Heat remaining 1 tablespoon oil in a large skillet over medium-high heat. Sauté mushrooms and onion until softened, about 5 minutes. Add flour to mushroom mixture and stir to thicken. Add water and tomato sauce and mix until smooth.

5. Pour tomato and mushroom mixture over meatballs. Cover and cook on low 3–4 hours. Serve warm.

Calories 350

PER SERVING

Fat 18g
Sodium 320mg
Carbohydrates 22g
Fiber 1g
Sugar 2g
Protein 23g

RICE AND SLOW COOKING

When making rice in a slow cooker, use converted rice (not instant) and it will come out light and fluffy. You can also add vegetables and spices to the rice for an easy meal.

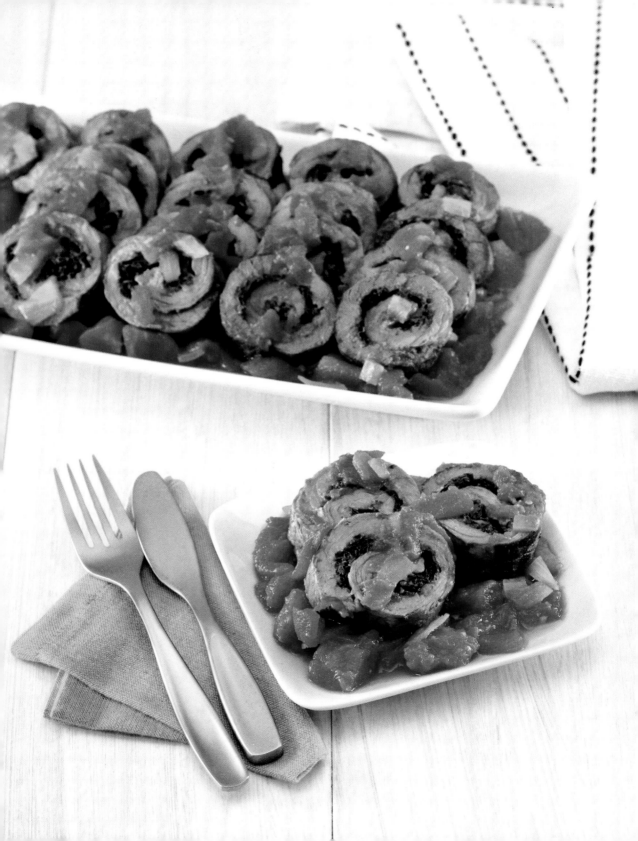

Braciola

Braciola is an Italian dish made of thin slices of meat that are filled and rolled up into a spiral shape. It tastes rich but doesn't contain too many calories. Look for steaks that are approximately ⅛" thick, 8"–10" long, and 5" wide to make this dish.

SERVES 8

½ teaspoon olive oil

½ cup diced onions

2 cloves garlic, peeled and minced

1 (32-ounce) can diced tomatoes

8 (2.5-ounce) very thin-cut round steaks

4 teaspoons bread crumbs

4 teaspoons grated Parmesan cheese

8 stalks rapini, stems cut off

1. Heat oil in a large skillet over medium-high heat. Sauté onions and garlic until onions are soft, about 5 minutes.

2. Place mixture in a 6-quart oval slow cooker. Add tomatoes and stir to combine.

3. Place steaks flat on a tray and sprinkle with bread crumbs and Parmesan. Place a bunch of rapini leaves on one end of each steak. Roll each steak lengthwise, so that the rapini filling is wrapped tightly. It should look like a spiral.

4. Place in the large skillet, seam-side down. Cook for 1 minute over medium-high heat to brown. Use tongs to carefully flip steaks and cook the other side for 1 minute.

5. Place each roll in a single layer on top of sauce mixture in slow cooker. Cover and cook on low 1–2 hours or until steaks are cooked through. Serve immediately.

Calories 180

PER SERVING

Fat 9g
Sodium 330mg
Carbohydrates 8g
Fiber 3g
Sugar 3g
Protein 17g

Spanish Beef Stew

This hearty stew is perfect for a cold day. For extra flavor use wrinkled Turkish olives (or other Mediterranean olives) instead of standard stuffed olives.

SERVES 8

1 tablespoon olive oil

2 cloves garlic, peeled and sliced

1 medium onion, peeled and sliced

3 slices bacon, cut into 1" pieces

1 pound stew beef, cubed

3 large Roma tomatoes, diced

1 bay leaf, crumbled

1/4 teaspoon sage

1/4 teaspoon marjoram

1/2 teaspoon paprika

1/2 teaspoon curry powder

1 teaspoon salt

2 tablespoons white wine vinegar

1 cup beef stock

1/2 cup white wine

4 medium potatoes, peeled and sliced

1/3 cup pitted sliced green olives

2 tablespoons chopped fresh parsley

1   Spray a 4- to 5-quart slow cooker with nonstick cooking spray. Heat oil in a large skillet over medium heat. Sauté garlic, onion, bacon, and beef until bacon and beef are done and onion is softened, about 7–8 minutes. Drain and transfer meat mixture to slow cooker.

2   Add tomatoes, bay leaf, sage, marjoram, paprika, curry powder, salt, vinegar, stock, and wine to slow cooker. Cover and cook on low 5 hours.

3   Add potatoes, olives, and parsley to slow cooker and cook 1 hour more. Serve warm.

Calories 160

PER SERVING

Fat 6g
Sodium 510mg
Carbohydrates 12g
Fiber 1g
Sugar 1g
Protein 16g

Grilled Burgers Stuffed with Cheese

This dish is often called biftekia in Greece. These flavorful burgers will take a backyard barbecue up a notch! Make sure to seal the edges of the biftekia well once you have folded them over in order to avoid having the melted stuffing leaking out into your barbecue. You can also use a combination of lamb and veal or just veal if you prefer.

SERVES 6

1 pound ground lamb

1 medium onion, peeled and grated

1 large egg

1/2 cup bread crumbs

1 1/2 tablespoons finely chopped fresh parsley

1/2 tablespoon dried oregano

1 tablespoon dried thyme

1/2 teaspoon freshly ground black pepper

1/2 teaspoon salt

1 1/2 tablespoons extra-virgin olive oil, divided

1/2 pound sliced kefalograviera or feta cheese

1. In a large bowl, use hands to combine lamb, onion, eggs, bread crumbs, parsley, oregano, thyme, pepper, salt, and 1 tablespoon oil into a single cohesive mass.

2. Take a tennis ball–sized piece of lamb mixture; roll between palms to form a smooth, compact ball.

3. Spread a piece of parchment paper over cutting board; flatten ball into a thin patty, about 1/4" thick. Try to ensure a uniform thickness.

4. Place a piece of cheese on top of flattened patty. Be sure to leave space around edges of cheese to ensure you can pinch meat closed around cheese. Take up farther edge of parchment paper; bring up and toward you to fold meat patty over cheese. Pinch overlapping edges of meat together well; use parchment paper to form patty around cheese. Repeat steps until you have six patties.

5. Preheat a gas or charcoal grill to medium-high heat. Brush outside of each patty with remaining 1/2 tablespoon oil. Grill about 6–7 minutes per side, or until done. Serve immediately.

Calories 270

PER SERVING

Fat 20g
Sodium 510mg
Carbohydrates 8g
Fiber 0g
Sugar 2g
Protein 16g

Short Ribs of Beef with Red Wine

Use your favorite dry red wine in this succulent beef dish that won't push you over your daily calorie count. Serve it on polenta or mashed potatoes to absorb the rich sauce.

SERVES 6

1½ pounds short ribs of beef, excess fat trimmed

1 tablespoon ground cumin

1 teaspoon dried thyme

½ teaspoon onion powder

½ teaspoon garlic powder

½ teaspoon salt

1 teaspoon freshly ground black pepper

1 tablespoon olive oil

2 large red onions, peeled and chopped

12 large plum tomatoes, chopped

1 cup dry red wine

4 cups vegetable broth

1 Season ribs with cumin, thyme, onion powder, garlic powder, salt, and pepper.

2 Heat oil over medium-high heat in a Dutch oven, and sear ribs on both sides until browned, about 5 minutes per side. Place ribs in a 6-quart slow cooker.

3 Add onions to Dutch oven and sauté for 2 minutes. Add tomatoes and sauté for 1 minute more. Add wine and deglaze the Dutch oven. Reduce heat to low and let wine reduce by half, about 10 minutes. Add broth and bring to a simmer.

4 Pour wine mixture over ribs. Cover and cook on low 6–8 hours. If you want sauce to thicken up, remove cover from slow cooker and turn on high 15 minutes before serving.

Calories 270

PER SERVING

Fat 14g
Sodium 630mg
Carbohydrates 13g
Fiber 3g
Sugar 7g
Protein 24g

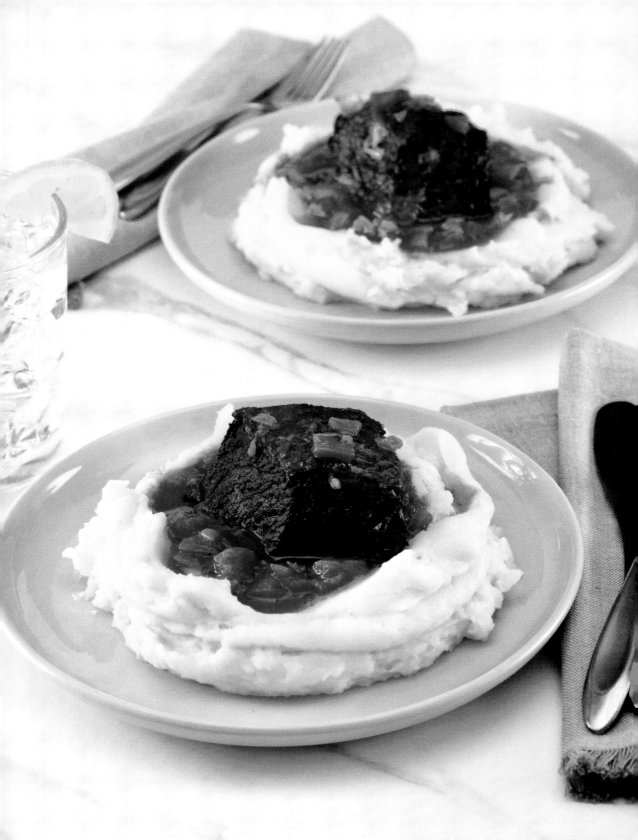

Seared Veal Medallions

This quick and easy dish is a great boost of protein and flavor. Feel free to try different varieties of mushrooms and olives to use what you have on hand and/or suit your palate. The low-calorie arugula provides calcium, vitamin C, vitamin A, and folate.

SERVES 6

2 tablespoons olive oil, divided

1½ pounds veal cutlets

½ teaspoon salt

1½ teaspoons freshly ground black pepper, divided

1 pound mushrooms, sliced

6 cloves garlic, peeled and minced

4 cups torn arugula

½ cup dry red wine

½ cup beef broth

¼ cup pitted chopped olives

1. Heat 1 tablespoon oil in a large skillet over medium-high heat. Season cutlets with salt and ½ teaspoon pepper, then sauté for 1 minute per side. Remove cutlets from pan and keep warm.

2. Reduce heat to medium and add remaining 1 tablespoon oil. Add mushrooms, garlic, and arugula; quickly sauté for 2 minutes. Add wine and cook for 1 minute, then add broth. Simmer for 10 minutes more.

3. Transfer mushroom mixture to a serving platter. Top with cutlets. Sprinkle with olives and remaining 1 teaspoon pepper before serving.

Calories 210

PER SERVING

Fat 9g
Sodium 450mg
Carbohydrates 5g
Fiber 1g
Sugar 2g
Protein 28g

Lemon Verbena Rack of Lamb

Lamb works wonderfully with lemon verbena, but you can always use lemon thyme in a pinch. Either way, the bright flavor of lemon adds a unique flavor dimension. Roasted potatoes are a wonderful side for this easy rack of lamb dish.

SERVES 8

2 (2-pound) racks lamb, silver skin removed and tied

¼ cup extra-virgin olive oil

2 cloves garlic, peeled and crushed

1 tablespoon Dijon mustard

1 teaspoon sweet paprika

1 tablespoon honey

2 teaspoons grated lemon zest

2 tablespoons chopped fresh parsley

2 tablespoons fresh lemon verbena leaves

2 teaspoons fresh thyme leaves

1 teaspoon salt

1 teaspoon freshly ground black pepper

1. Place lamb in a medium baking dish. In a food processor, add oil, garlic, mustard, paprika, honey, lemon zest, parsley, lemon verbena, and thyme, and process until well incorporated. Pour marinade over lamb and rub it all over to coat. Cover and marinate 1 hour at room temperature. Season with salt and pepper.

2. Preheat broiler. Place lamb on a medium baking sheet lined with parchment paper and roast under the broiler for 5 minutes.

3. Preheat oven to 450°F and roast lamb for 25 minutes, or until the internal temperature reads 135°F. If you prefer the meat well done, roast lamb for a few minutes more.

4. Tent lamb with foil and let rest 5 minutes before serving.

Calories 320

PER SERVING

Fat 23g
Sodium 360mg
Carbohydrates 0g
Fiber 0g
Sugar 0g
Protein 27g

GET THE BUTCHER'S HELP

Ask your butcher to trim the rack of lamb and remove its silver skin. He or she will then tie the lamb into a crown rack, which will save you some preparation time.

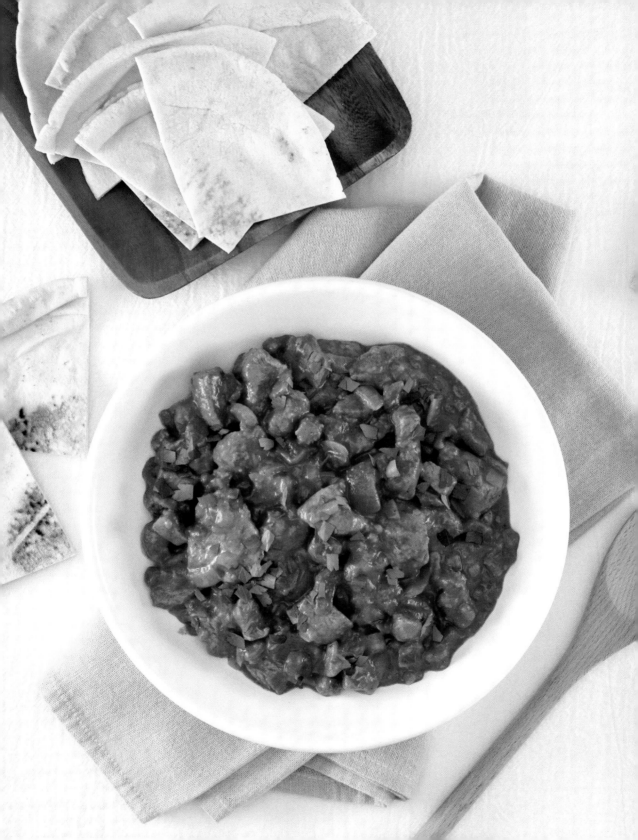

Ginger Tomato Lamb

You can substitute beef or pork for lamb in this recipe if you wish. Serve with triangles of fresh pita bread for a filling and protein-packed meal.

SERVES 8

2 tablespoons unsalted butter

2 pounds boneless lamb, cubed

1 medium onion, peeled and chopped

1 clove garlic, peeled and minced

3 tablespoons all-purpose flour

1½ tablespoons curry powder

2 large tomatoes, chopped

1 (1") piece ginger, peeled and grated

½ teaspoon salt

¼ cup water

1. Spray a 4- to 5-quart slow cooker with nonstick cooking spray. Heat butter in a large skillet over medium heat. Sauté lamb until slightly browned, about 8 minutes. Transfer meat to slow cooker; set aside pan with juices.

2. Add onion and garlic to pan used for lamb and sauté over medium heat until onion is tender, about 10 minutes. Stir in flour and curry powder. Continue cooking until thickened, about 5 minutes.

3. Add onion and garlic mixture, tomatoes, ginger, salt, and water to slow cooker. Cover and cook on low 4–5 hours. Serve warm.

Calories 340

PER SERVING

Fat 26g
Sodium 220mg
Carbohydrates 6g
Fiber 1g
Sugar 2g
Protein 20g

Braised Lamb Shoulder

The herbs and spices impart a unique flavor combination in this slow-roasted dish. Serve with rice, spaghetti, or potatoes.

SERVES 6

½ cup extra-virgin olive oil

1½ pounds lamb shoulder, cut into small piece with bones

½ cup hot water

2 cups fresh tomatoes, diced and sieved

2 bay leaves

4 cloves garlic, peeled and minced

1 cinnamon stick

1 tablespoon dried thyme

⅛ teaspoon salt

⅛ teaspoon freshly ground black pepper

1. Heat olive oil in a large pot over medium-high heat. Add lamb and brown on all sides, about 5 minutes.

2. Add water, tomatoes, bay leaves, garlic, cinnamon, thyme, salt, and pepper. Cover and bring to a boil, then reduce heat to medium-low.

3. Simmer for 1½ hours, stirring occasionally. Serve warm.

Calories 400

PER SERVING

Fat 36g
Sodium 110mg
Carbohydrates 3g
Fiber 1g
Sugar 2g
Protein 16g

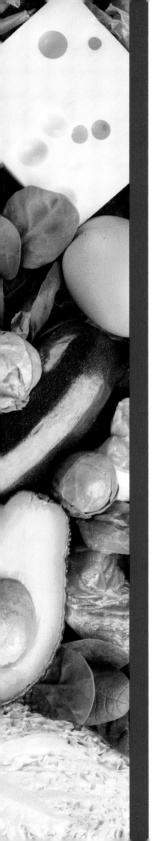

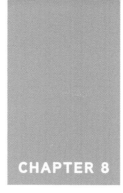

CHAPTER 8

Pork Main Dishes

Lean pork can provide a source of protein for the Mediterranean diet. The dishes in this chapter will help you upgrade the standard pork chop meal with many tasty options, from sausage to meatballs to casseroles. Whether you prefer the spicy Sausage and Peppers or the mild Fennel Chops, you're sure to find a recipe that helps you meet your calorie goals and tastes delicious too.

Paprika Meatballs

These flavorful meatballs can be served with skewers as a finger food or over pasta as a main dish. They are excellent with fresh angel hair pasta or eaten in a sandwich for lunch the next day.

SERVES 12

1 pound ground veal	3 large eggs	1/2 cup 1% milk
1 pound ground pork	1 tablespoon paprika	2 tablespoons vegetable oil
1 clove garlic, peeled and minced	1 teaspoon salt	2 large plum tomatoes, diced
1/4 pound shredded mozzarella cheese	1 cup bread crumbs	1 cup tomato sauce

1. In a large bowl, combine veal, pork, garlic, and mozzarella. Add eggs, paprika, salt, bread crumbs, and milk; mix well. Form mixture into twelve equal-sized balls.

2. Spray a 4- to 5-quart slow cooker with nonstick cooking spray. Heat vegetable oil in a large skillet over medium heat. Working in batches, brown meatballs on all sides, about 1 minute per side. Place meatballs on a tray lined with paper towels to absorb excess oil.

3. Arrange meatballs in slow cooker. Pour tomatoes and tomato sauce over meatballs. Cover and cook on low 3–4 hours. Serve hot.

Calories 260

PER SERVING

Fat 17g
Sodium 440mg
Carbohydrates 8g
Fiber 1g
Sugar 1g
Protein 20g

PASTA AND SLOW COOKING

Pasta is a great addition to slow-cooked meals, but it shouldn't be added until your dish is almost ready. Add uncooked pasta to slow cooker about 1 hour before serving.

Italian Pork with Cannellini Beans

This incredibly simple-to-make one-dish meal is packed with flavor. Cannellini beans are an excellent source of fiber, and contain folate and iron as well. For instructions on how to roast your own garlic, see the sidebar with the Wax Beans with Roasted Garlic, Capers, and Parsley recipe in Chapter 5.

SERVES 6

1½ pounds pork loin

1 (28-ounce) can crushed tomatoes

1 medium onion, peeled and minced

2 tablespoons capers

1 head roasted garlic, peels removed

1 (15-ounce) can cannellini beans, drained and rinsed

2 teaspoons Italian seasoning

1. Place pork, tomatoes, onion, capers, and roasted garlic into a 4- to 5-quart ungreased slow cooker. Cover and cook on low 7–8 hours.

2. One hour before serving, add cannellini beans and Italian seasoning.

Calories 310

PER SERVING

Fat 11g
Sodium 430mg
Carbohydrates 23g
Fiber 3g
Sugar 7g
Protein 30g

Sausage and Peppers

This is a one-pan dish of spicy sausages, onions, peppers, and tomatoes called spetsofai in Greece. The bell peppers provide a healthy dose of beta carotene and vitamin A. Use your favorite sausage and enjoy this dish with crusty bread and a dry red wine.

SERVES 8

3 tablespoons extra-virgin olive oil, divided

4 (5") fresh pork sausages

4 medium hot banana peppers, cored and skins pierced

2 large red or yellow bell peppers, seeded and sliced

2 medium onions, peeled and sliced

4 cloves garlic, peeled and minced

2 large ripe tomatoes, peeled and grated

1/2 teaspoon salt

1/2 teaspoon freshly ground black pepper

2 teaspoons dried oregano

1 Heat 2 tablespoons oil in a large skillet over medium-high heat for 30 seconds. Add sausages and brown, 2–3 minutes per side. Remove sausages from skillet and set aside.

2 Add banana peppers to skillet and fry on all sides until just brown, about 1–1½ minutes per side. Remove banana peppers and slice. Set aside.

3 Add bell peppers, onions, garlic, and tomatoes to skillet. Bring mixture to a boil and then reduce heat to medium-low. Season with salt and black pepper. Slice sausages and return with banana peppers to skillet. Cover and cook for 15–20 minutes or until sauce thickens.

4 Uncover skillet and add oregano. Drizzle remaining 1 tablespoon oil over sausage mixture. Serve hot.

Calories 120

PER SERVING

Fat 9g
Sodium 250mg
Carbohydrates 9g
Fiber 3g
Sugar 5g
Protein 4g

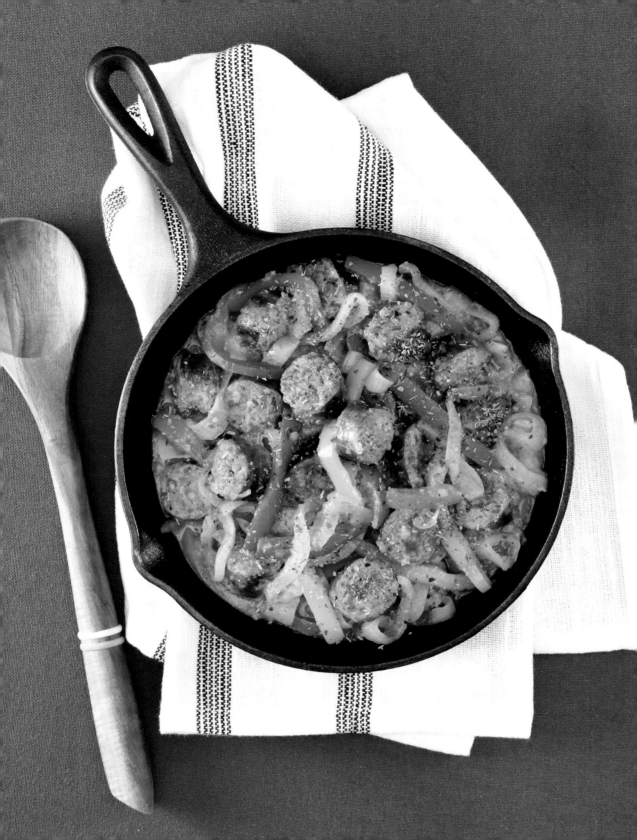

Pork Roast with Prunes

Pork pairs wonderfully with fruit, and this recipe is no exception. The prunes add richness to the pork along with fiber to help aid digestion and fullness. This is a perfect weekend dish in cooler weather.

SERVES 6

1½ pounds lean pork roast, excess fat removed

1 medium onion, peeled and diced

2 cloves garlic, peeled and minced

¾ cup pitted prunes

½ cup water

½ teaspoon freshly ground black pepper

¼ teaspoon salt

⅛ teaspoon ground nutmeg

⅛ teaspoon ground cinnamon

Place all ingredients into a 4- to 5-quart slow cooker. Cover and cook on low 8 hours. Serve warm.

Calories 320

PER SERVING

Fat 20g
Sodium 270mg
Carbohydrates 14g
Fiber 2g
Sugar 6g
Protein 20g

Pork Skewers

This dish, often called souvlaki in Greece, comes together very quickly once the marinade is done. For extra nutrition, add chopped vegetables to the skewers. You can also try this marinade with other meats, such as beef shoulder or lamb shoulder.

SERVES 8

1 large onion, peeled and grated

3 cloves garlic, peeled and minced

1 teaspoon salt

$3/4$ teaspoon freshly ground black pepper

$1/4$ cup plus 3 tablespoons vegetable oil, divided

4 teaspoons dried oregano, divided

2 pounds boneless pork butt, fat trimmed and cut into 1" cubes

2 large lemons, cut into wedges

1 In a large bowl, whisk onion, garlic, salt, pepper, $1/4$ cup vegetable oil, and 2 teaspoons oregano. Add pork and toss to coat. Refrigerate pork at least 5 hours or overnight. Bring pork to room temperature before grilling.

2 Put pork onto wooden or metal skewers; each skewer should hold four pieces.

3 Preheat a gas or charcoal grill to medium-high heat. When grill is ready, dip a clean tea towel in remaining 3 tablespoons vegetable oil and wipe the grill's surface. Place skewers on the grill and cook for 3–4 minutes per side or until pork is cooked through.

4 Sprinkle pork with the remaining 2 teaspoons oregano and serve with lemon wedges.

Calories 260

PER SERVING

Fat 21g
Sodium 330mg
Carbohydrates 2g
Fiber 1g
Sugar 1g
Protein 18g

SOAK WOODEN SKEWERS FIRST

When using wooden skewers for grilling, always soak them in water for 2 hours before spearing the food. Soaking the skewers prevents them from burning when placed on the grill.

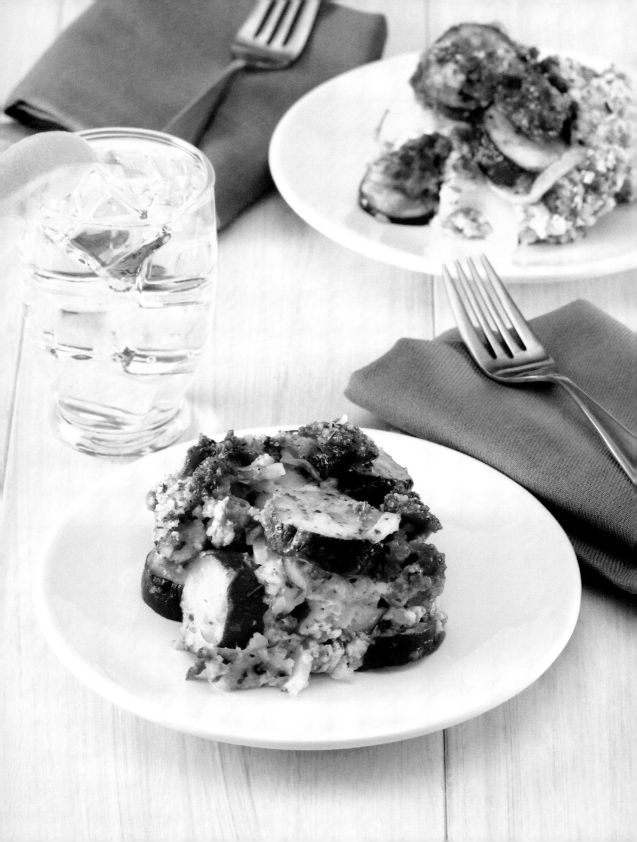

Zucchini and Sausage Casserole

Yes, you can still enjoy a hearty casserole while counting calories! Serve this casserole on a bed of mixed greens with a fruit salad on the side.

SERVES 6

1 pound mild pork sausage, casings removed

1¼ cups grated Parmesan cheese

½ teaspoon salt

½ teaspoon freshly ground black pepper

1 teaspoon dried mint

½ teaspoon dried oregano

½ teaspoon dried basil

2 large eggs, beaten

1 cup whole milk

3 medium zucchini, trimmed and sliced into ½" rounds

1 small onion, peeled and sliced

1. In a large skillet, brown sausage over medium heat about 10 minutes until no longer pink. Drain fat from skillet and set sausage aside. Discard fat.

2. In a large bowl, whisk together Parmesan, salt, pepper, mint, oregano, and basil.

3. In another large bowl, whisk together eggs and milk.

4. Spray a 4- to 5-quart slow cooker with nonstick cooking spray. Place one third of zucchini over the bottom of the slow cooker. Add one third of onion over zucchini. Add one third of cooked sausage over onion. Add one third of milk mixture over sausage. Lastly, add one third of Parmesan mixture over everything. Repeat layers two more times, ending with Parmesan mixture.

5. Cover, vent lid with a chopstick, and cook on low 6 hours or on high 3 hours. Cut into squares to serve.

Calories 370

PER SERVING

Fat 27g
Sodium 1,100mg
Carbohydrates 12g
Fiber 2g
Sugar 6g
Protein 21g

Caper Pork

Here is your opportunity to use capers in a dish other than chicken piccata. The capers in this vegetable-packed recipe give the pork a refreshing zing.

SERVES 8

2 tablespoons olive oil

2 pounds pork loin, cut into 8 equal-sized pieces

1 medium onion, peeled and sliced

4 stalks celery, ends trimmed and sliced

2 medium carrots, peeled and sliced

3 cloves garlic, peeled and minced

1 cup tomato sauce

6 pitted quartered black olives

1/4 cup dry white wine

1 tablespoon capers

1. Spray a 4- to 5-quart slow cooker with nonstick cooking spray. Heat oil in a large skillet over medium-high heat. Sauté pork until lightly browned, about 5 minutes per side. Remove pork from pan and place in prepared slow cooker, leaving meat juices in the pan.

2. In the same skillet, sauté onion, celery, carrots, and garlic over high heat for 5 minutes. Transfer vegetable mixture to slow cooker. Pour tomato sauce over vegetables and pork. Cover and cook on low 6–8 hours.

3. Half an hour before serving, add olives, wine, and capers to slow cooker.

Calories 360

PER SERVING

Fat 25g
Sodium 230mg
Carbohydrates 11g
Fiber 3g
Sugar 5g
Protein 23g

FINDING BLACK OLIVES

Many grocery stores now carry a wide assortment of olives. Try the giant black olives and the small wrinkled ones. You might discover varieties of olives that you didn't even know existed. Once you taste them, chances are you'll forsake the pimiento-stuffed versions in jars and use those other varieties in your cooking instead.

Fennel Chops

These chops are very savory thanks to their distinct fennel flavor. To complement them, all you need is a simple side of wild rice, some fresh bread, or steamed vegetables.

SERVES 6

2 cloves garlic	6 (6-ounce) pork chops	1 tablespoon fennel seeds
1/2 teaspoon salt	2 tablespoons olive oil	1 cup white wine

1. Crush garlic and salt into a paste and rub over chops.

2. Heat oil in a large skillet over medium-high heat. Sauté chops until lightly browned, about 5 minutes per side.

3. Spray a 4- to 5-quart slow cooker with nonstick cooking spray. Put chops, pan drippings, fennel seeds, and wine into slow cooker. Cover and cook on low 3–4 hours. Serve immediately.

Calories 330

PER SERVING

Fat 20g
Sodium 290mg
Carbohydrates 1g
Fiber 0g
Sugar 0g
Protein 35g

Sautéed Pork Medallions and Potatoes

Potatoes can get a bad reputation in dieting circles, but that's probably because they're often prepared in unhealthy ways. The roasted potatoes here contain fiber and potassium. Leaving the skins on provides an extra boost of magnesium too.

SERVES 6

1½ tablespoons olive oil

4 cloves garlic, peeled and minced

1½ pounds pork tenderloin, sliced into thin medallions

2 pounds russet potatoes, thinly sliced

2 tablespoons chopped fresh oregano

½ teaspoon freshly ground black pepper

2 tablespoons pitted minced black olives

1 Heat oil in a large skillet over medium heat. Sauté garlic for 30 seconds and then add pork and potatoes. Sprinkle with oregano and pepper.

2 Reduce heat to medium-low, cover, and cook about 20 minutes.

3 Flip potatoes and pork and cook, uncovered, for 10 minutes more. Transfer to a serving platter. Top with olives before serving.

Calories 270

PER SERVING

Fat 6g
Sodium 80mg
Carbohydrates 28g
Fiber 2g
Sugar 1g
Protein 27g

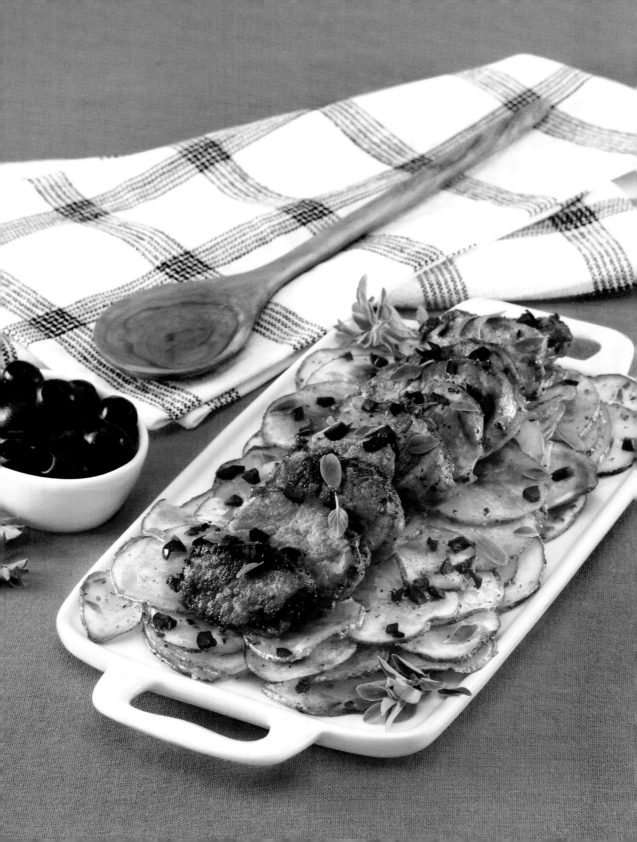

Greek-Style Meatballs and Artichokes

Mediterranean flavors abound in this dish thanks to the lemon, artichokes, and olives. Serve it with an orzo pilaf for a satisfying meal that still allows you to stay on track with your calorie goals.

SERVES 12

2 thin slices white sandwich bread, crumbled

1/2 cup 1% milk

2 3/4 pounds lean ground pork

2 cloves garlic, peeled and minced

1 large egg

1/2 teaspoon grated lemon zest

1/4 teaspoon freshly ground black pepper

16 ounces frozen artichoke hearts, defrosted

3 tablespoons fresh lemon juice

2 cups low-sodium chicken broth

3/4 cup frozen chopped spinach, defrosted

1/3 cup pitted sliced Greek olives

1 tablespoon minced fresh oregano

1. Preheat oven to 350°F.

2. In a shallow saucepan, combine bread and milk. Cook over low heat until milk is absorbed, about 1 minute. Transfer to a large bowl and add pork, garlic, egg, lemon zest, and pepper. Mix until all ingredients are evenly distributed. Roll into 1" balls.

3. Line two medium baking sheets with parchment paper. Place meatballs in a single layer on baking sheets. Bake for 15 minutes and then place on a tray lined with paper towels.

4. Add meatballs to a 6-quart slow cooker. Add artichokes, lemon juice, broth, spinach, olives, and oregano. Cover and cook on low 6–8 hours. Serve warm.

Calories 290

PER SERVING

Fat 19g
Sodium 240mg
Carbohydrates 9g
Fiber 3g
Sugar 1g
Protein 22g

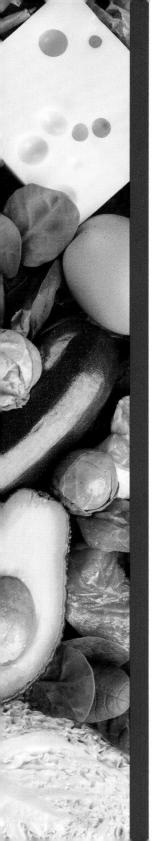

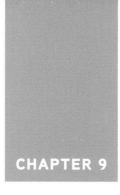

CHAPTER 9

Seafood and Fish Main Dishes

Thanks to its prime location, foods from the sea play a huge part of the Mediterranean diet. Fish provides a healthy source of protein with few calories. With the wide variety of tastes and textures available from seafood, you're sure to find several types that appeal to your palate. From the simplicity of Olive Oil–Poached Cod to the bolder flavors in Salmon with Anchovy Caper Vinaigrette, the choices are endless! Try to cook fish shortly after you purchase it for best flavor and freshness.

Olive Oil–Poached Cod

Poaching cod in olive oil produces a succulent, delicate fish that will wow your family or guests even though it is simple to make. Serve this poached fish on a bed of wild rice or alongside steamed vegetables.

SERVES 4

3 cups extra-virgin olive oil

4 (6-ounce) fresh cod fillets, skins removed

1/2 teaspoon salt

2 tablespoons fresh lemon juice

1 tablespoon grated lemon zest

1 Choose a pot that will just fit the fillets and fill it with oil. Bring oil to a temperature of 210°F. Adjust heat to keep the temperature at 210°F while poaching fillets.

2 Carefully place fillets in the oil and poach until opaque in color, about 6 minutes. Carefully remove fish from oil and place on a serving plate. Sprinkle fillets with salt.

3 Spoon some of the warm oil over fillets and then drizzle with lemon juice. Sprinkle with lemon zest and serve immediately.

Calories 290

PER SERVING

Fat 18g
Sodium 380mg
Carbohydrates 1g
Fiber 0g
Sugar 0g
Protein 30g

WHAT IS POACHING?

Poaching is a gentle cooking method for fish, meat, chicken, and eggs. The item is submerged in a liquid (oil, broth, or water) and cooked at a low temperature. This method helps keep food moist while giving it the flavor of the cooking liquid.

Spinach-Stuffed Sole

This impressive dish is easy to make but looks very sophisticated.
Choose any flat fish fillet as a substitute for sole. Serve these fillets
on a bed of Braised Lentils (see recipe in Chapter 5).

SERVES 4

4 tablespoons extra-virgin olive oil, divided

4 scallions, ends trimmed and sliced

1 pound frozen spinach, defrosted and drained

3 tablespoons chopped fresh fennel fronds or tarragon leaves

$3/4$ teaspoon salt, divided

$1/2$ teaspoon freshly ground black pepper, divided

4 (6-ounce) sole fillets, skins removed

2 tablespoons plus $1 1/2$ teaspoons grated lemon zest, divided

1 teaspoon sweet paprika

1. Preheat oven to 400°F. Line a baking sheet with parchment paper.

2. Heat 1 tablespoon oil in a medium skillet over medium heat for 30 seconds. Add scallions and cook for 3–4 minutes. Remove scallions from skillet and place in a medium bowl. Cool to room temperature.

3. Add spinach and fennel to scallions and mix well. Season with $1/4$ teaspoon salt and $1/4$ teaspoon pepper.

4. Rub fillets with 1 tablespoon oil and sprinkle with 2 tablespoons lemon zest. Season fillets with remaining $1/2$ teaspoon salt and $1/4$ teaspoon pepper and sprinkle with paprika.

5. Divide spinach filling among fillets. Roll up each fillet, starting from the widest end. Use two toothpicks to secure each fillet. Place rolled fillets on the baking sheet and drizzle remaining 2 tablespoons oil over them.

6. Bake for 15–20 minutes. Remove toothpicks and sprinkle fillets with remaining $1 1/2$ teaspoons lemon zest. Serve immediately.

Calories 290

PER SERVING

Fat 18g
Sodium 1,030mg
Carbohydrates 7g
Fiber 4g
Sugar 1g
Protein 26g

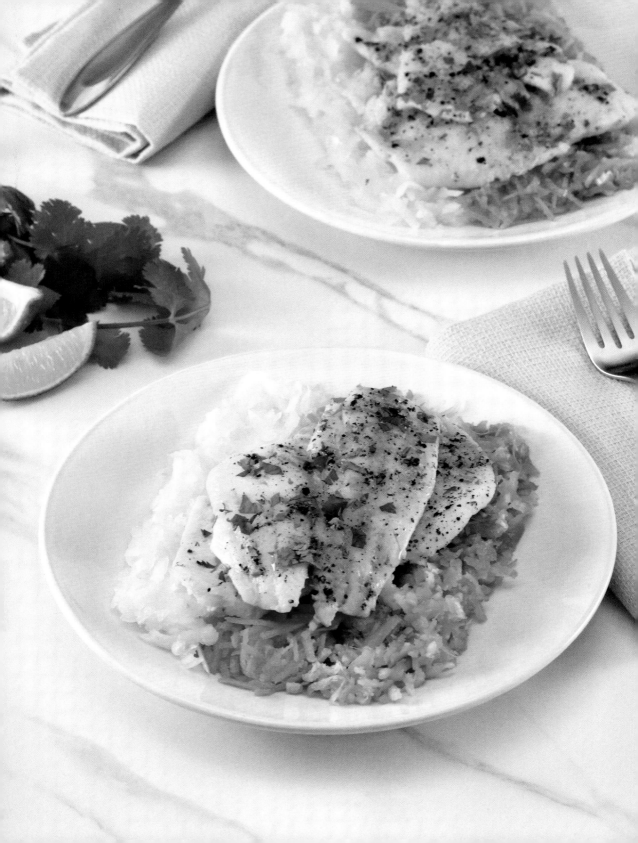

Lime-Poached Flounder

Lime brings out the delicate flavor of the fish and complements the zip of the cilantro. Try this fresh-tasting but very low-calorie dish when the weather is hot.

SERVES 6

1 medium leek, trimmed and sliced

1/2 bunch fresh cilantro, leaves separated from stems

1 1/2 pounds flounder fillets

1 3/4 cups fish stock or fat-free chicken broth

2 tablespoons fresh lime juice

1/2 teaspoon grated lime zest

1/2 teaspoon salt

1/2 teaspoon freshly ground black pepper

2 medium yellow onions, peeled and grated

2 large carrots, peeled and grated

2 stalks celery, ends trimmed and grated

2 tablespoons extra-virgin olive oil

1. In a large skillet, place leek slices and cilantro stems, then lay fillets on top.

2. Add stock, lime juice, lime zest, salt, and pepper. Bring to a slow boil over medium-high heat. Reduce heat to medium-low, cover, and cook for 7–10 minutes until fillets are thoroughly cooked. Remove from heat. Strain off and discard liquid.

3. To serve, lay grated onions, carrots, and celery in separate strips on a serving platter. Top with fillets, drizzle with olive oil, and sprinkle with cilantro leaves.

Calories 160

PER SERVING

Fat 7g
Sodium 620mg
Carbohydrates 9g
Fiber 2g
Sugar 4g
Protein 15g

USING FROZEN FISH

Don't fret if you don't have fresh fish available in your area. Using a quality fish frozen at sea is perfectly fine. In fact, sometimes the frozen fish is fresher than the fresh!

Salmon with Anchovy Caper Vinaigrette

Salmon is rich in healthy omega-3 fatty acids, so it's a good fish to work into your meal rotations. If you see multicolored heirloom tomatoes in your market, try them in this dish.

SERVES 6

1 tablespoon olive oil

6 (5-ounce) salmon fillets

6 anchovy fillets

1 large beefsteak tomato, thinly sliced

1/2 cup plain low-fat Greek yogurt

1/4 cup capers

3 tablespoons finely chopped fresh chives

1. Preheat oven to 375°F. Pour oil into a large roasting pan and then place salmon in the pan. Place anchovies on top and roast for 10 minutes.

2. Remove from oven. Slice salmon and place on plates. Top salmon with tomato slices. Dollop yogurt on tomato slices, then sprinkle with capers and chives. Serve immediately.

Calories 230

PER SERVING

Fat 9g
Sodium 310mg
Carbohydrates 3g
Fiber 1g
Sugar 2g
Protein 32g

Grilled Grouper Steaks

Grouper has a firm meat that doesn't dry out easily and holds up well on the grill. Serve this fish with a heaping spoonful of salsa and roasted potatoes.

SERVES 4

1/4 cup extra-virgin olive oil

1 tablespoon grated lemon zest

1/2 cup dry white wine

1/2 teaspoon chopped fresh rosemary leaves

4 (1/3-pound) grouper steaks, rinsed and dried

3 tablespoons vegetable oil

1/2 teaspoon salt

1. In a medium baking dish, whisk olive oil, lemon zest, wine, and rosemary. Add fish and toss to combine. Cover with plastic and refrigerate 1 hour. Allow fish to return to room temperature 30 minutes before grilling.

2. Preheat a gas or charcoal grill to medium-high heat. When grill is ready, dip a clean tea towel in vegetable oil and wipe the grill surface. Sprinkle fish with salt on both sides and grill for 5–6 minutes per side. Serve hot.

Calories 150

PER SERVING

Fat 3g
Sodium 370mg
Carbohydrates 0g
Fiber 0g
Sugar 0g
Protein 29g

Oven-Poached Bass with Kalamata Chutney

Bass is a low-carb, high-protein fish that will keep you full without being full of calories. Kalamata olives have a very distinctive flavor and add a touch of saltiness to this dish.

SERVES 6

1 medium shallot, peeled and chopped

1 stalk celery, ends trimmed and chopped

1/2 teaspoon freshly ground black pepper

1 1/2 pounds bass fillet

1/2 cup dry white wine

1 cup fish stock or clam juice

1/4 cup pitted chopped Kalamata olives

2 cloves garlic, peeled and minced

1/4 teaspoon grated lemon zest

1. Preheat oven to 400°F. Place shallot and celery in the bottom of a large baking dish; sprinkle with pepper. Place fish on top and add wine and stock. Cover and bake for 15–20 minutes.

2. For the chutney, mix olives, garlic, and lemon zest in a small bowl.

3. Remove fish from the cooking liquid and serve with a spoonful of chutney.

Calories 150

PER SERVING

Fat 4g
Sodium 250mg
Carbohydrates 3g
Fiber 0g
Sugar 1g
Protein 22g

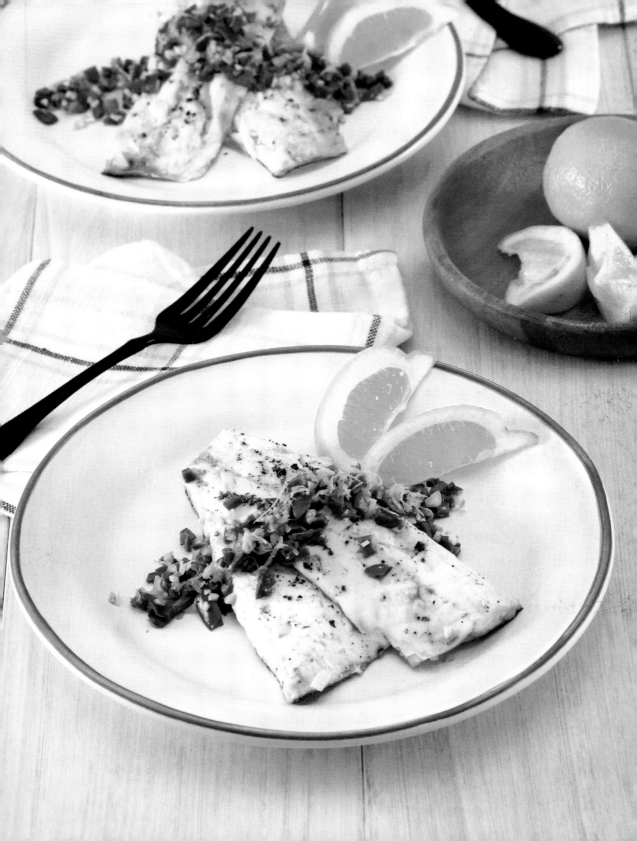

Mussels Marinara

Mussels contain a lot of protein, as well as zinc, omega-3 fatty acids, and folate. Serve these mussels on a bed of pasta and have bread on hand to soak up the sauce.

SERVES 6

1 tablespoon olive oil

2 small shallots, peeled and minced

3 cloves garlic, peeled and minced

6 medium plum tomatoes, roughly chopped

3 pounds mussels

1 cup dry red wine

1/2 cup fish stock or clam juice

1/4 teaspoon crushed red pepper

1 teaspoon dried oregano

1. Heat oil in a large saucepan over medium heat. Add shallots, garlic, and tomatoes and sauté for 5 minutes.

2. Add mussels, wine, stock, crushed red pepper, and oregano. Cook, stirring occasionally, until mussels open, about 3–5 minutes. Serve immediately.

Calories 240

PER SERVING

Fat 7g
Sodium 700mg
Carbohydrates 13g
Fiber 2g
Sugar 4g
Protein 29g

Braised Cuttlefish

Cuttlefish are a type of mollusk with ten legs similar to octopus and squid. If you haven't cooked cuttlefish before, don't be intimidated. The tentacles, eyes, skin, and beak of the cuttlefish need to be removed along with the ink sack and central bony cartilage, but most fish markets will do this for you.

SERVES 6

1/3 cup extra-virgin olive oil

2 large onions, peeled and diced

3 cloves garlic, peeled and pressed or finely chopped

2 pounds cuttlefish, cut into strips

1 cup red wine

2 cups tomatoes, minced

2 tablespoons finely chopped fresh parsley

1 teaspoon dried marjoram

1 bay leaf

1/8 teaspoon salt

1/8 teaspoon freshly ground black pepper

1. Heat oil in a large skillet over medium-high heat. Add onions and sauté until soft, about 3 minutes.

2. Add garlic and sauté for 30 seconds or so before adding (drained) fish. Continue to sauté and stir continuously until fish starts to turn a yellowish color, about 6–8 minutes.

3. Add wine and cook for 10 minutes more, stirring regularly.

4. Add tomatoes, parsley, marjoram, bay leaf, salt, and pepper. Cover and simmer over medium-low until sauce has thickened and fish is tender, about 90 minutes. Add 1/2–1 cup water to pan if liquid thickens before fish has softened sufficiently.

5. Serve warm with fresh bread.

Calories 300

PER SERVING

Fat 14g
Sodium 750mg
Carbohydrates 10g
Fiber 1g
Sugar 5g
Protein 26g

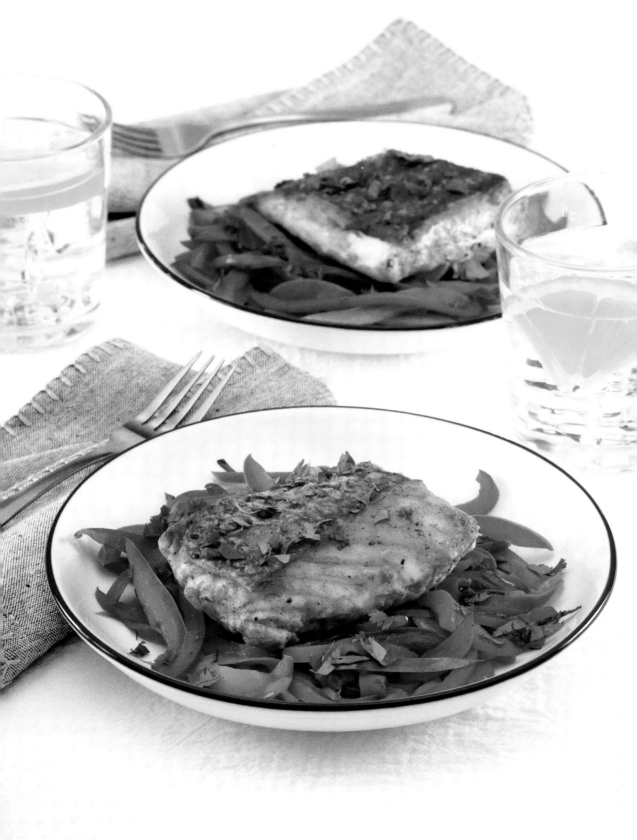

Red Snapper with Peppers and Vinegar

The tartness of the vinegar and the sweetness of the peppers perfectly complement the unique flavor of red snapper. Red snapper is an excellent source of protein, selenium, potassium, and vitamin B_{12}.

SERVES 6

$\frac{1}{4}$ cup all-purpose flour

1 tablespoon curry powder

$\frac{1}{2}$ teaspoon freshly ground black pepper

$1\frac{1}{2}$ pounds red snapper

1 tablespoon olive oil

1 medium red bell pepper, seeded and thinly sliced

1 medium green bell pepper, seeded and thinly sliced

1 tablespoon cider vinegar

$\frac{1}{4}$ cup chopped fresh cilantro

1. In a medium shallow dish, mix flour, curry powder, and black pepper together. Dredge fish in flour mixture.

2. Heat oil in a large skillet over medium-high heat. Cook fish for 5 minutes per side.

3. Add bell peppers and vinegar. Reduce heat to medium-low and simmer for 5 minutes more until fish flakes easily with a fork. Sprinkle with cilantro before serving.

Calories 160

PER SERVING

Fat 4g
Sodium 95mg
Carbohydrates 6g
Fiber 1g
Sugar 1g
Protein 23g

Stovetop Fish

Due to the heat of the summer months in Mediterranean countries, dishes like this are common, as you do not have to use an oven that will add heat to the kitchen. The simple flavors in this recipe allow the gentle fish flavor to shine.

SERVES 6

3 tablespoons extra-virgin olive oil

4 cloves garlic, peeled and minced

1 pound tomatoes, peeled and minced

6 fresh mint leaves, finely chopped

1/8 teaspoon salt

1/8 teaspoon freshly ground black pepper

1 tablespoon dried oregano

1/2 cup water

2 pounds white fish fillets

1 1/2 cups chopped fresh parsley

1. Heat oil in a large skillet over medium-high heat. Add garlic and quickly sauté, about 1 minute. Add tomatoes, mint, salt, pepper, and oregano. Bring to a boil and let simmer for 10 minutes, until thickened.

2. Add water and continue to simmer for 3–4 minutes more.

3. Place fish in skillet and simmer for 15 minutes. Do not stir; simply shake pan gently from time to time to avoid sticking.

4. Garnish fish with parsley and serve immediately with rice.

Calories 290

PER SERVING

Fat 16g
Sodium 260mg
Carbohydrates 6g
Fiber 1g
Sugar 3g
Protein 30g

Grilled Sea Bass

The secret to successfully grilling sea bass is to not overcook it, so make sure to check the fish on the grill for flakiness and remove it quickly when it is done. Sea bass offers a ton of protein with relatively few calories.

SERVES 4

4 (1½-pound) whole sea bass

⅛ teaspoon freshly ground black pepper

⅛ teaspoon salt

¼ cup fresh lemon juice

¼ cup extra-virgin olive oil

1 teaspoon dried oregano

1 cup finely chopped fresh parsley

2 lemons, sliced

1½ tablespoons vegetable oil

1. Using a sharp knife, cut several diagonal slits on both sides of each fish. Sprinkle with salt and pepper, including inside the cavity.

2. In a small bowl, mix lemon juice, olive oil, and oregano. Divide mixture and set half aside.

3. Stuff each fish with parsley and several lemon slices.

4. Brush both sides of each fish liberally with ½ olive oil and lemon mixture.

5. Preheat a gas or charcoal grill to medium heat. When grill is ready, dip a clean tea towel in vegetable oil and wipe the grill's surface. Place fish on grill and close the cover.

6. Grill for 15 minutes, until fish flakes easily. Brush with remaining olive oil and lemon mixture and serve hot.

Calories 360

PER SERVING

Fat 23g
Sodium 200mg
Carbohydrates 2g
Fiber 1g
Sugar 1g
Protein 34g

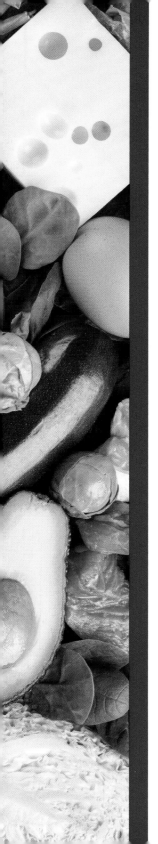

CHAPTER 10

Vegetarian Main Dishes

Keeping an emphasis on vegetables will help you stay on track with your calorie goals, since most vegetables are naturally low in calories. In this chapter, vegetables are the star of the show! These dishes are still hearty, filling, and full of flavor—just because they're vegetarian doesn't mean they're bland, light meals! Try working in a vegetarian meal or two every week to boost your intake of nutrient-rich foods. From the colorful Chickpea Salad with Roasted Red Peppers and Green Beans to the classic Stuffed Eggplant, these vegetarian dishes will satisfy your taste buds and your waistline.

Zucchini Pie with Herbs and Cheese

This is a fantastic savory pie. Serve it with a simple green salad for a perfect brunch or lunch dish. Zucchini are naturally low in calories, though this dish won't taste like it!

SERVES 12

½ cup extra-virgin olive oil

12 scallions, ends trimmed and finely chopped

4 medium zucchini, 3 diced and 1 thinly sliced into rounds

½ teaspoon salt

5 large eggs

1 cup self-rising flour

1 teaspoon baking powder

1 cup strained plain Greek yogurt

1 cup crumbled feta cheese

1 cup grated kasseri or Gouda cheese

1 teaspoon freshly ground black pepper

2 teaspoons sweet paprika, divided

1 cup chopped fresh dill

1. Preheat oven to 350°F. Heat oil in a large skillet over medium heat for 30 seconds. Add scallions, diced zucchini, and salt. Cook about 20 minutes to soften vegetables and evaporate half of their released liquids. Take skillet off heat and set aside.

2. In a large bowl, whisk eggs for 2 minutes. Stir in flour and baking powder. Stir in yogurt. Stir in cheeses and softened vegetables. Stir in pepper, 1½ teaspoons paprika, and dill.

3. Pour mixture into a large, deep, greased baking dish. Top with zucchini rounds and sprinkle with remaining ½ teaspoon paprika.

4. Place the dish on the middle rack and bake for 1 hour. Allow pie to cool about 15 minutes before cutting into slices and serving.

Calories 260

PER SERVING

Fat 18g
Sodium 460mg
Carbohydrates 13g
Fiber 2g
Sugar 4g
Protein 11g

CHEESE SUBSTITUTIONS

Kasseri cheese is a Greek sheep's milk cheese that is often served on its own. If you can't find kasseri, Gruyère or Gouda works just as well.

Pasta with Cherry Tomatoes, Cheese, and Basil

*This classic and simple dish is as colorful as it is tasty. Use any
ripe chopped tomato if you can't find cherry tomatoes.*

SERVES 8

2 tablespoons extra-virgin olive oil

1 pint cherry tomatoes, halved

3 1/2 teaspoons salt, divided

1/4 teaspoon freshly ground black pepper

6 cloves garlic, peeled and minced

1 pound broad egg noodles

1 cup diced Halloumi cheese

1 cup sliced fresh basil

1 1/2 cups crumbled feta cheese

1/2 cup plain low-fat Greek yogurt

1/2 teaspoon crushed red pepper

1. Heat oil in a large skillet over medium heat for 30 seconds. Add tomatoes, 1/2 teaspoon salt, and black pepper. Cover skillet and cook for 5 minutes. Uncover and mash tomatoes slightly to release their juices. Add garlic and cook for 10 minutes or until sauce thickens.

2. Fill a large pot two-thirds with water and place over medium-high heat. Add remaining 3 teaspoons salt and bring water to a boil. Add noodles and cook for 6–7 minutes or until al dente. Reserve 1/4 cup cooking water and drain pasta.

3. Add pasta to sauce and stir to combine. If the sauce is a little thin or dry, stir in reserved pasta water. Stir in Halloumi and basil.

4. In a medium bowl, combine feta, yogurt, and crushed red pepper. Mash everything together with a fork. Add feta mixture to pasta and stir until sauce is creamy.

5. Serve immediately.

Calories 370

PER SERVING

Fat 14g
Sodium 692mg
Carbohydrates 45g
Fiber 1g
Sugar 4g
Protein 17g

MORE ON BASIL

The word *basil* in Greek is *basilikos*, which means "king." In the Mediterranean, there's no doubt that basil is the king of herbs. There are many varieties to be found, so try as many as you can to find your favorite.

Greek Pita

Pita bread offers a perfect pocket for fillings. Serve these simple but flavorful sandwiches with a green salad for a light vegetarian lunch or dinner when you'd rather not turn on the oven.

SERVES 6

6 large loaves pita bread

2 medium cucumbers, peeled and diced

1 large red onion, peeled and thinly sliced

1/4 cup chopped fresh oregano

1/2 cup crumbled feta cheese

1 tablespoon olive oil

1/2 teaspoon freshly ground black pepper

1. Cut a slit into each pita and stuff with cucumber, onion, oregano, and feta.

2. Drizzle with oil and sprinkle with black pepper before serving.

Calories 240

PER SERVING

Fat 6g
Sodium 440mg
Carbohydrates 39g
Fiber 1g
Sugar 2g
Protein 8g

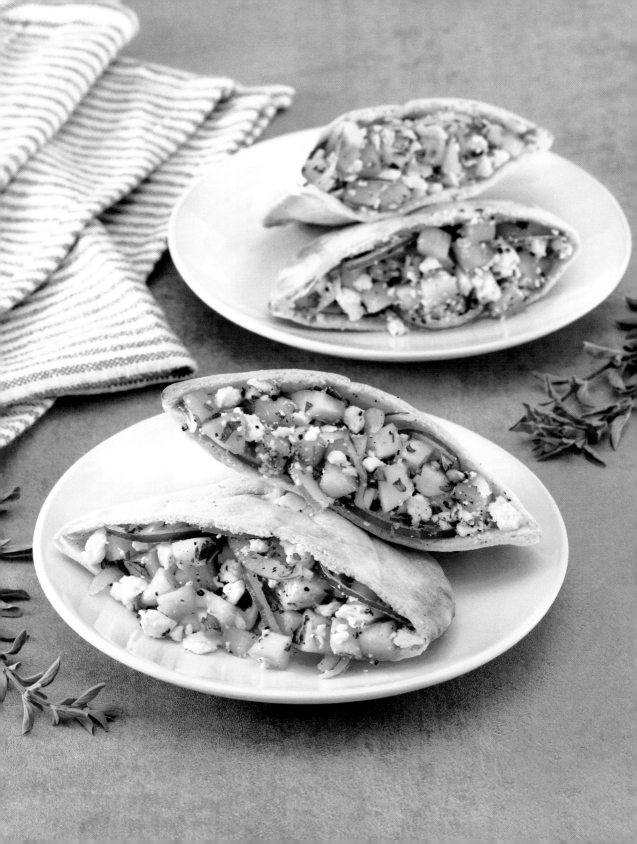

Artichokes à la Polita

Recipes with the term polita *refer to dishes from Constantinople/Istanbul. This stewlike dish features lots of vegetables for a nutritional boost to your day.*

SERVES 8

¼ cup extra-virgin olive oil

2 medium onions, peeled and sliced

4 medium potatoes, peeled and cut into thirds

3 large carrots, peeled and cut into 2" pieces

1 tablespoon tomato paste

12 medium artichokes, outer layers peeled, trimmed, halved, and chokes removed

1 teaspoon salt

¾ teaspoon freshly ground black pepper

1 cup frozen (defrosted) or fresh peas

½ cup chopped fresh dill

1 large lemon, cut into wedges

1 Heat oil in a large pot over medium-high heat. Stir in onions, potatoes, and carrots. Reduce heat to medium and cover. Simmer for 15–20 minutes.

2 Add tomato paste, artichokes, salt, pepper, and enough water to cover. Bring to a boil, cover pot, and reduce temperature to medium. Cook for 10 minutes or until artichokes are tender.

3 Gently stir in peas and dill. Take pot off heat and allow peas to cook for 5 minutes more. Serve hot with lemon wedges.

Calories 240

PER SERVING

Fat 8g
Sodium 520mg
Carbohydrates 38g
Fiber 13g
Sugar 6g
Protein 10g

Bulgur-Stuffed Zucchini

The bulgur, tomatoes, parsley, mint, and lemon in the stuffing are reminiscent of a Middle Eastern tabbouleh. Bulgur is a great alternative to traditional rice because it contains much more fiber and folate.

SERVES 6

3 small zucchini

2 teaspoons extra-virgin olive oil

1 medium shallot, peeled and diced

3 cloves garlic, peeled and minced

1 cup bulgur wheat

2 medium leeks, trimmed and thinly sliced

1/2 cup dry white wine

3 cups vegetable broth

1 medium tomato, chopped

1 teaspoon grated lemon zest

1/2 cup chopped fresh mint

1/4 cup chopped fresh parsley

1. Preheat oven to 375°F. Cut zucchini in half lengthwise and use a spoon to hollow out each half. Discard insides. Place halves in a medium microwave-safe dish, cut-side down. Pour in just enough water to cover the bottom of the dish. Microwave 1–2 minutes on high. Set aside to cool slightly.

2. Heat oil in a medium stockpot over medium heat. Add shallot, garlic, and bulgur. Cook, stirring constantly until slightly brown, about 5 minutes. Add leeks and cook for 3 minutes more. Pour in wine and let reduce, about 1 minute.

3. Add broth and simmer for 15 minutes until bulgur is thoroughly cooked. Remove from heat and stir in tomato, lemon zest, mint, and parsley.

4. Spoon bulgur mixture into zucchini halves and place on a large baking sheet. Bake until zucchini is reheated, about 5–8 minutes. Serve warm.

Calories 150

PER SERVING

Fat 2g
Sodium 280mg
Carbohydrates 28g
Fiber 5g
Sugar 5g
Protein 5g

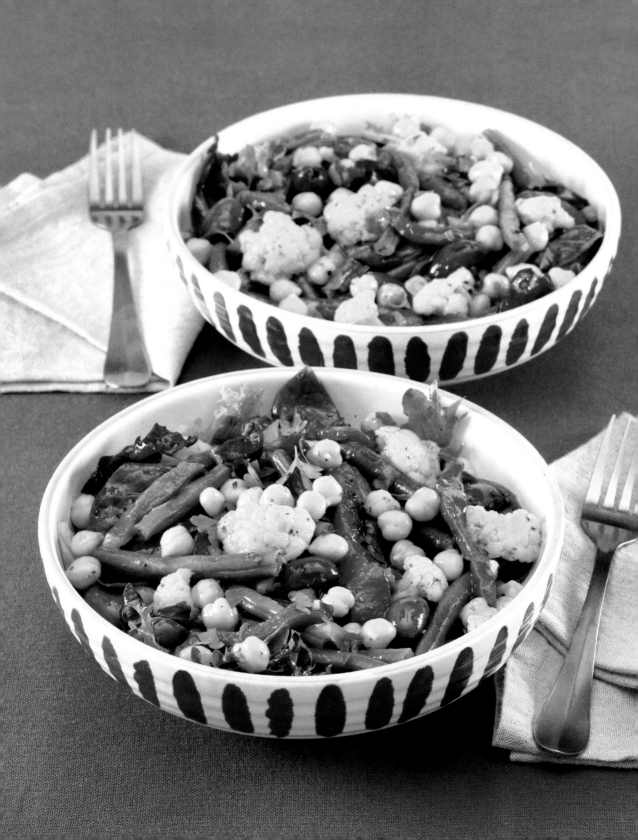

Chickpea Salad with Roasted Red Peppers and Green Beans

This light salad is a great option when you're attending a warm weather potluck event. Try using a combination of red, green, yellow, or orange peppers for a more colorful salad. For instructions on how to blanch vegetables, see the sidebar with the Roasted Vegetables with Beans recipe in this chapter.

SERVES 6

3 cloves garlic, peeled and minced

1 teaspoon Dijon mustard

2 tablespoons red wine vinegar

3/4 teaspoon salt, divided

1/2 teaspoon freshly ground black pepper, divided

1/2 cup extra-virgin olive oil

1 (15-ounce) can chickpeas, drained and rinsed

1 pound green beans, trimmed and blanched for 5–6 minutes

2 large roasted red peppers (see the sidebar), sliced

1 cup pickled jarred or canned cauliflower florets, halved

5 ounces spring mix salad greens

1/4 cup chopped fresh parsley

2 teaspoons dried oregano

12 pitted Kalamata olives

1. In a large bowl, whisk garlic, mustard, vinegar, 1/2 teaspoon salt, and 1/4 teaspoon black pepper. Slowly whisk in oil until it is well incorporated.

2. Add chickpeas, beans, roasted peppers, and cauliflower. Toss to coat.

3. Add greens, parsley, oregano, olives, and remaining 1/4 teaspoon salt and 1/4 teaspoon pepper. Toss to combine ingredients and serve immediately.

Calories 370

PER SERVING

Fat 25g
Sodium 730mg
Carbohydrates 31g
Fiber 9g
Sugar 9g
Protein 8g

HOW TO MAKE YOUR OWN ROASTED PEPPERS

To make roasted red peppers, grill 6 large red bell peppers on a clean grill after wiping surface with olive oil. Char pepper on all sides. Place the peppers in a bowl and cover tightly with plastic wrap. Cool 20 minutes. Remove charred skins and discard. Slit the peppers in half; remove and discard the seeds and stem.

Stuffed Eggplant

This wonderful dish—called imam bayildi in Greece or Turkey—can be served on its own or as a side dish. If you can't find allspice berries, you can instead use up to ½ teaspoon of ground allspice, or an equivalent mixture of cinnamon, nutmeg, and cloves.

SERVES 6

6 medium eggplants, stems removed

3 teaspoons salt, divided

½ cup extra-virgin olive oil, divided

4 medium onions, peeled and thinly sliced, divided

1 medium green bell pepper, seeded and sliced

6 whole allspice berries, wrapped tightly in thin cheesecloth

1 (14-ounce) can whole tomatoes, hand crushed

1 teaspoon freshly ground black pepper

10 cloves garlic, peeled and thinly sliced

2 teaspoons dried oregano

1 teaspoon fresh thyme leaves

½ cup chopped fresh parsley

2 medium tomatoes, thinly sliced

1 Preheat oven to 375°F. Cut eggplants in half lengthwise and use a spoon to hollow out each half, leaving a ¼" thick shell. Reserve flesh. Evenly sprinkle 1½ teaspoons salt over hollowed-out shells and place flesh-side down on a large plate. Coarsely chop scooped-out flesh, place in a strainer, and sprinkle with ½ teaspoon salt. Set aside.

2 Heat ¼ cup oil in a large skillet over medium-high heat for 30 seconds. Add two-thirds onions. Add green peppers and allspice. Cook for 1 minute. Reduce heat to medium and cover. Cook for 10–15 minutes or until vegetables soften.

3 Stir in scooped-out eggplant flesh, crushed tomato, and remaining 1 teaspoon salt and black pepper. Cook for 20–30 minutes or until reduced to a thick, chunky sauce. Remove allspice. Adjust seasoning with more salt and pepper, if necessary. Stir in garlic, oregano, thyme, and parsley.

4 Place the inverted shells upright in a large, shallow baking dish. Pat the insides dry with a paper towel. Spoon vegetable sauce evenly into each shell. Pour enough hot water around eggplants to come halfway up the sides.

Calories 270

PER SERVING

Fat 15g
Sodium 960mg
Carbohydrates 34g
Fiber 13g
Sugar 16g
Protein 5g

5 Cover each eggplant with tomato slices and remaining one-third onions. Drizzle the remaining ¼ cup oil evenly over eggplants. Bake for 45–60 minutes or until most of the water has evaporated and the tops are golden brown. Serve warm.

THE FAINTING PRIEST

Imam bayildi, which means "fainting priest," is originally a Turkish dish, but it is also very popular in Greece. The story behind imam bayildi is that when a Muslim priest (or imam) tasted this dish of olive oil, sweet eggplant, and vegetables for the first time, he fainted because it was so delicious.

Pasta with Arugula and Brie

Try to find high-quality cheese and garlic for this recipe, since those ingredients really shine against the simple backdrop. Removing the rind from Brie is an optional step, depending on your personal preference. For instructions on how to roast your own garlic, see the sidebar with the Wax Beans with Roasted Garlic, Capers, and Parsley recipe in Chapter 5.

SERVES 8

6 cloves roasted garlic, peels removed

1 teaspoon salt

1 1/4 pounds pasta

5 ounces baby arugula

6 ounces roughly chopped Brie cheese

1 teaspoon extra-virgin olive oil

1 teaspoon freshly ground black pepper

1. Fill a large pot two-thirds with water and place it over medium-high heat. Add salt and bring water to a boil. Add pasta and cook for 6–7 minutes or until al dente. Drain pasta.

2. In a large bowl, toss all ingredients together until arugula wilts and cheese melts slightly. Serve hot.

Calories 350

PER SERVING

Fat 8g
Sodium 164mg
Carbohydrates 55g
Fiber 3g
Sugar 2g
Protein 14g

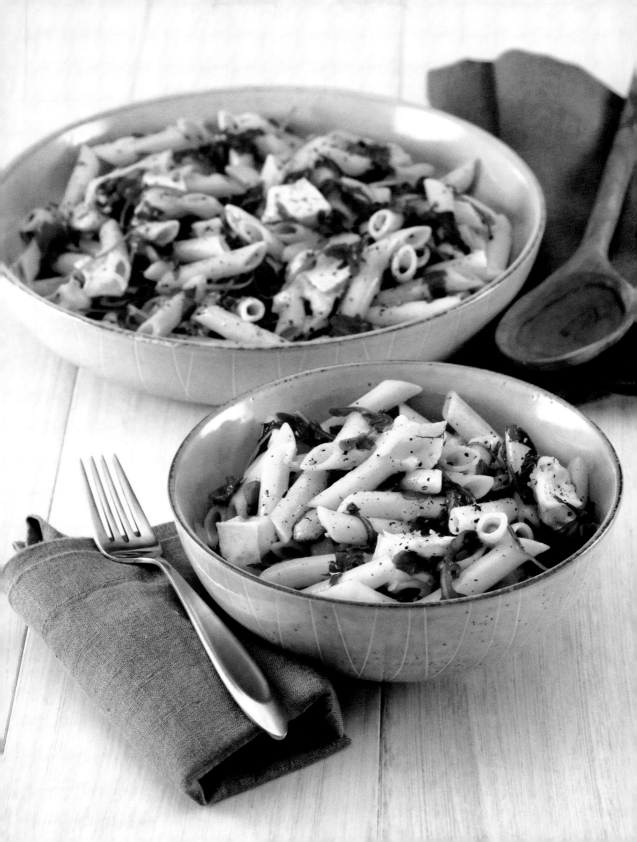

Roasted Vegetables with Beans

This dish is often called tourlou *in Greece, which means "mixed-up vegetables." Some crusty bread and a slab of feta cheese would pair nicely with this recipe.*

SERVES 6

3/4 cup extra-virgin olive oil, divided

2 large onions, peeled and sliced

6 cloves garlic, peeled and minced

2 teaspoons salt, divided

1 teaspoon freshly ground black pepper, divided

2 large zucchini, sliced

2 long Japanese eggplants, sliced

6 medium plum or Roma tomatoes, chopped

1 cup chopped fresh parsley

1 tablespoon fresh thyme leaves

1 cup chopped fresh basil

1 pound green beans, trimmed and blanched, cooled to room temperature

1 Preheat oven to 375°F. Heat 1/2 cup oil in a large skillet over medium heat for 30 seconds. Add onions, garlic, 1/4 teaspoon salt, and 1/4 teaspoon pepper. Cook mixture for 6–7 minutes or until onions are translucent. Spread onion mixture evenly over the bottom of a medium casserole dish.

2 In a medium bowl, combine zucchini, eggplant, tomatoes, parsley, thyme, and the remaining 1/4 cup oil. Season with remaining 1 3/4 teaspoon salt and remaining 3/4 teaspoon pepper. Top onion mixture with vegetables, and stir to combine the ingredients.

3 Cover dish with aluminum foil and bake for 1 hour. Remove foil and sprinkle top with basil. Allow the tourlou to cool for 10 minutes before serving. Vegetables can be cooled completely, stored in the refrigerator, and reheated the next day.

4 To serve the tourlou, arrange the beans on the bottom of a plate or serving platter, and then top them with the warm vegetable mixture (including juices).

Calories 380

PER SERVING

Fat 29g
Sodium 800mg
Carbohydrates 26g
Fiber 9g
Sugar 14g
Protein 6g

BLANCHING VEGETABLES

Blanching refers to a cooking technique in which vegetables are boiled briefly in salted water; then, the cooking process is stopped quickly by plunging the vegetables in ice water. This technique keeps vegetables tender and preserves their bright natural colors.

Zucchini Blossoms with Rice

Zucchini blossoms are the edible flowers of the zucchini plant. This dish is a lovely, unique one to serve at a special event. A feta and yogurt sauce would pair nicely with this dish.

SERVES 6

30 zucchini blossoms, stemmed and small outer leaves removed

½ cup extra-virgin olive oil, divided

1 large onion, peeled and chopped

2 cloves garlic, peeled and minced

2 medium tomatoes, peeled and grated

1 cup Arborio rice, rinsed

¼ cup dry white wine

2 medium zucchini, 1 trimmed and grated, 1 trimmed and thinly sliced

½ cup chopped fresh parsley

2 tablespoons chopped fresh mint

2 tablespoons chopped fresh dill

2 teaspoons salt

1 teaspoon freshly ground black pepper

2 cups hot vegetable stock

1. Place blossoms in a large bowl with warm water for 10 minutes. Rinse blossoms under cool tap water and set upside-down to dry.

2. Heat ¼ cup oil in a large skillet over medium heat for 30 seconds. Add onion, garlic, and tomatoes. Simmer for 5–7 minutes or until onion is translucent.

3. Stir in rice, wine, and grated zucchini. Simmer for 15 minutes more. If most of the cooking liquid dries up, add 2 tablespoons hot water. Stir in parsley, mint, and dill. Take skillet off heat. Season with salt and pepper.

4. Preheat the oven to 350°F. Line bottom of a large baking dish with sliced zucchini. Gently open a blossom and insert 1 teaspoon of rice mixture. Fold petals inward to seal filling and place blossom in the dish. Repeat this process for remaining blossoms. Arrange blossoms in a taut, circular pattern in the dish.

5. Add stock and drizzle blossoms with remaining ¼ cup oil. Place an inverted (ovenproof) plate over blossoms and cover the dish. Bake for 30–40 minutes or until rice has cooked. Serve warm or at room temperature.

Calories 340

PER SERVING

Fat 20g
Sodium 810mg
Carbohydrates 35g
Fiber 4g
Sugar 5g
Protein 6g

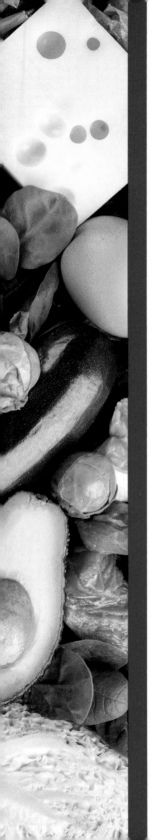

CHAPTER 11

Desserts

Even when you're counting calories, you can often fit in a treat or two on occasion. The recipes in this chapter can help you satisfy your sweet tooth without overindulging. Plus, many dishes offer nutritional value as well, thanks to the nuts, fruits, and honey that those in the Mediterranean region use to sweeten their desserts naturally. Try the decadent Cypriot Cookies for a special celebration, or the Almond Tangerine Bites for a no-bake fresh-tasting treat. Finish off your meal with one of these recipes as you imagine yourself looking out onto the lovely blue Mediterranean Sea!

Stuffed Figs

Figs are a sweet dessert, but do not contain the processed sugars present in many American desserts. A nutritional bonus: Figs contain antioxidants and fiber! Purchase dried Kalamata string figs if you can find them, as they are larger and sweeter than most other commercially available varieties.

SERVES 4

12 dried figs, stalks trimmed

24 walnut halves

2 tablespoons thyme honey

2 tablespoons sesame seeds

1. Slice the side of each fig and open with fingers.

2. Stuff two walnut halves inside each fig and fold closed.

3. Arrange figs on a serving platter. Drizzle with honey and sprinkle with sesame seeds to serve.

Calories 190

PER SERVING

Fat 9g
Sodium 10mg
Carbohydrates 27g
Fiber 4g
Sugar 21g
Protein 3g

Almond Tangerine Bites

This Greek almond treat originates from the island of Kérkyra (or Corfu), one of the Ionian Islands off the west coast of Greece. These light bites are just sweet enough and perfect for a warm night.

SERVES 24

2 cups raw almonds

5 medium tangerines, divided

1 cup brown sugar

Icing sugar, for dusting

1. Fill a large pot two-thirds with water and set over medium-high heat. Bring water to a boil and add almonds to blanch, about 1 minute. When almonds start floating to top, remove from water, drain, and peel.

2. Fill a second large pot two-thirds with water over medium-high heat. Bring water to a boil and add 3 tangerines to remove bitterness from rind, about 5 minutes.

3. Squeeze juice from remaining 2 tangerines and set aside; discard skins.

4. Peel 3 boiled tangerines; discard pulp. In a blender, purée skins and blanched almonds until very finely ground.

5. In a large bowl, combine almond mixture with brown sugar.

6. Slowly add tangerine juice and mix well.

7. Roll small pieces of mixture into 24 walnut-sized balls using palms of hands. Set aside on wax paper to dry.

8. Dust balls lightly with icing sugar before serving.

Calories 100

PER SERVING

Fat 5g
Sodium 0mg
Carbohydrates 13g
Fiber 2g
Sugar 11g
Protein 2g

ALMONDS: THE GREEK NUT

The ancient Romans referred to the almond as the "Greek nut" because the almond tree had its origins in Asia Minor (modern-day Turkey).

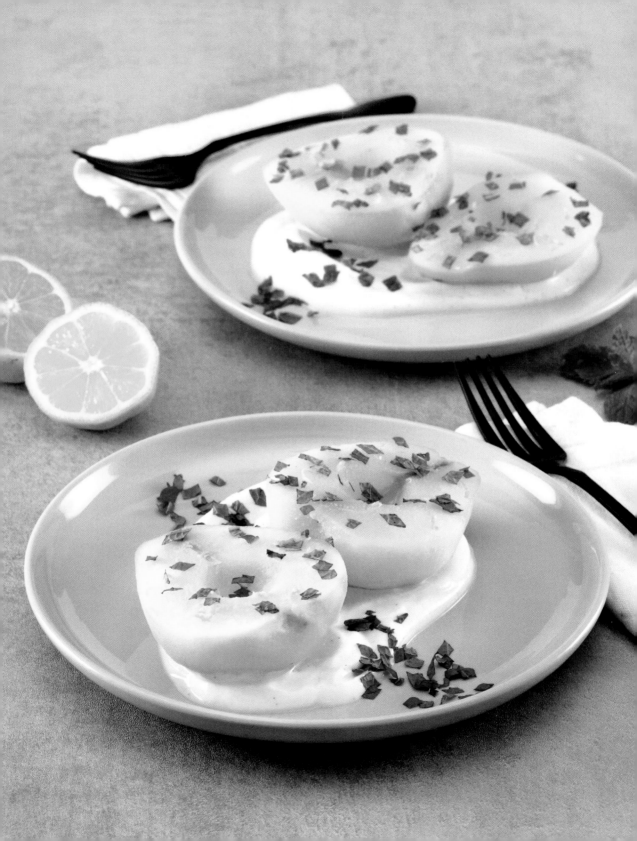

Roasted Pears

Featuring fruits as dessert is a key facet of the Mediterranean diet. The advantages are twofold—you can enjoy a low-calorie dessert and get nutritional benefits as well. Try your favorite light wine as you savor this recipe, or try it with pear cider or eau-de-vie.

SERVES 6

6 medium pears, peeled, cored, and halved

1 cup sweet white wine

1 tablespoon grated lemon zest

1 teaspoon honey

3 ounces vanilla low-fat yogurt

¼ cup chopped fresh mint

1. Preheat oven to 375°F.

2. Place pears cut-side down in a small roasting pan. Add wine, lemon zest, and honey. Cover and roast for 30 minutes. Uncover and roast for 10 minutes more.

3. Place a dollop of yogurt on each plate. Top with pear halves and sprinkle with mint.

Calories 120

PER SERVING

Fat 0g
Sodium 10mg
Carbohydrates 29g
Fiber 5g
Sugar 18g
Protein 2g

Café Frappé

Frappé is among the most popular drinks in Greece and is available at virtually all Greek cafés. Add a small shot of anise-flavored ouzo to your evening frappé!

SERVES 1

1 tablespoon instant coffee

1 teaspoon sugar

1 tablespoon room temperature water

½ cup cold water

2 tablespoons evaporated milk

1. In a cocktail shaker, add coffee, sugar, and water. Cover and shake vigorously for 30 seconds.

2. Pour mixture into a tall glass with a few ice cubes. Add enough cold water to almost fill the glass.

3. Add milk and serve immediately with a straw.

Calories 110

PER SERVING

Fat 2.5g
Sodium 45mg
Carbohydrates 19g
Fiber 0g
Sugar 7g
Protein 4g

Berries and Meringue

A perfect ending to a picnic, this meringue provides a sweet, light finish to any warm weather lunch. If you like, stir a few tablespoons of sugar into the berries about 15–30 minutes before serving.

SERVES 12

6 large egg whites
1/2 cup sugar

1/4 teaspoon cream
of tartar

2 cups fresh berries
(blackberries, blueberries,
raspberries, or a combination)

1. Preheat oven to 200°F. Line a large baking sheet with parchment paper or spray with nonstick cooking spray.

2. In a large copper or stainless steel bowl, beat egg whites, sugar, and cream of tartar until stiff. Drop egg white mixture onto baking sheet to form twelve small mounds. Bake for 1 1/2–1 3/4 hours, until dry, crispy, and lightly golden.

3. Place each meringue on a dessert plate. Top with berries.

Calories 50

PER SERVING

Fat 0g
Sodium 30mg
Carbohydrates 11g
Fiber 1g
Sugar 10g
Protein 2g

Sesame Snaps

These warmly flavored dessert bites can satisfy a sweet tooth without breaking your diet. Replace the orange zest with lemon zest if you prefer a lemon flavor for this light dessert.

SERVES 16

1 tablespoon unsalted butter	1/3 cup honey	1 1/3 cups toasted sesame seeds (see the sidebar)
2 cups sugar	1 teaspoon fresh lemon juice	
1/3 cup water	1/4 teaspoon sea salt	1 tablespoon grated orange zest

1. Grease a medium baking sheet with butter. In a medium heavy-bottomed pan, bring sugar, water, honey, lemon juice, and salt to a boil over medium-high heat. Continue cooking 10 minutes or until mixture turns into a deep amber-colored syrup.

2. Stir sesame seeds and orange zest into syrup. Remove pan from heat. Immediately pour syrup onto baking sheet. Quickly spread evenly around pan with a greased spatula.

3. Before syrup cools completely, score the top into serving pieces (squares or diamond shapes) with a greased knife. When syrup has cooled completely, remove it from pan with a spatula and cut into serving pieces.

4. Store in an airtight container.

Calories 170

PER SERVING

Fat 4.5g
Sodium 55mg
Carbohydrates 32g
Fiber 1g
Sugar 31g
Protein 2g

TOASTING SESAME SEEDS

Toasting sesame seeds is easy, but it requires some patience. Put sesame seeds in a dry frying pan over medium heat. Stir them constantly with a wooden spoon until they are toasted to your liking. Toasting can take up to 10 minutes, so be patient. Don't walk away from the pan because the seeds burn very quickly.

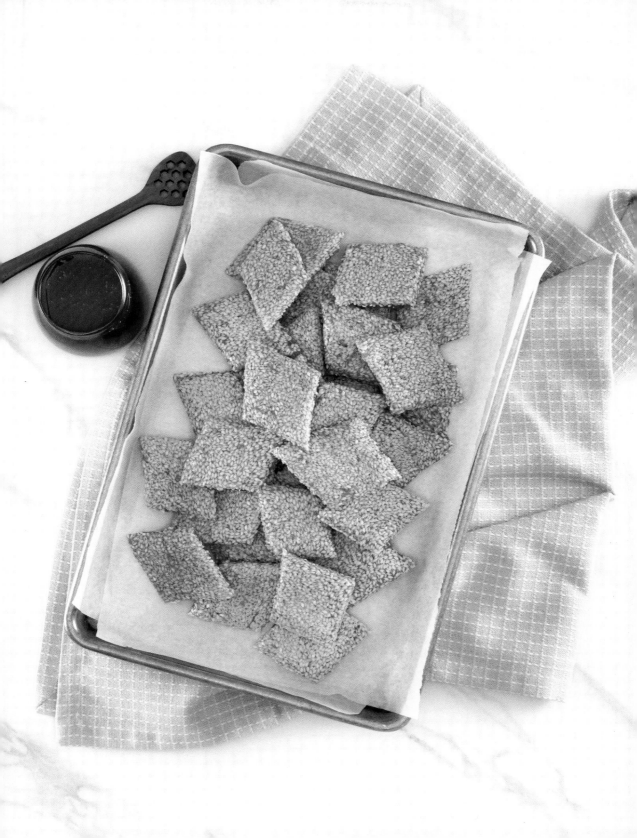

Honey Fritters

These fritters are often called loukoumades in Greece. Many recipes for loukoumades call for a boiled sugar-honey-water syrup bath, but in most cases, the honey is sweet enough on its own. You can also sprinkle the loukoumades with some crushed walnuts before serving. Loukoumades are best eaten on the same day they are made.

SERVES 35

1½ tablespoons active dry yeast

1½ cups lukewarm 1% milk or water, divided

4 cups all-purpose flour

½ teaspoon salt

3 cups vegetable oil for deep-frying

1 cup cold water

1 cup good-quality Greek honey

Ground cinnamon, for dusting

1. In a mixing bowl, dissolve yeast in 1 cup milk; cover bowl with cloth and let stand 10 minutes to allow yeast to rise.

2. Gently add flour and salt to mixing bowl in stages; continue to mix well.

3. Sparingly add remaining ½ cup milk while continually mixing. Add additional milk if necessary to ensure dough is soft and sticky. Dough should be soft enough to drop from a spoon.

4. Cover mixing bowl with cloth and place in a warm spot to rise, about 1–2 hours, or until dough has doubled in bulk and bubbles form on the surface.

5. When dough has risen, heat oil in a large, deep pan over medium-high heat. Working in batches, dip a measuring teaspoon into cold water and then scoop a small portion of dough. Drop each dollop of dough directly into pan, being sure to dip teaspoon in water in between to ensure that dough does not stick. If using fingers to remove dough from teaspoon, remember to wipe between each teaspoonful.

Calories 110

PER SERVING

Fat 2.5g
Sodium 40mg
Carbohydrates 20g
Fiber 1g
Sugar 8g
Protein 2g

6 Fry each batch until fritters puff up and achieve a golden brown color, about 3–4 minutes. Remove fritters from oil with slotted spoon and place on paper towels to absorb excess oil for 1–2 minutes.

7 Arrange fritters on a serving platter and drizzle honey to cover. Dust with cinnamon powder and serve immediately.

ARISTAEUS AND HONEY

According to Greek mythology, a lesser god by the name of Aristaeus was credited with teaching humanity husbandry and agriculture, including the art of beekeeping for honey.

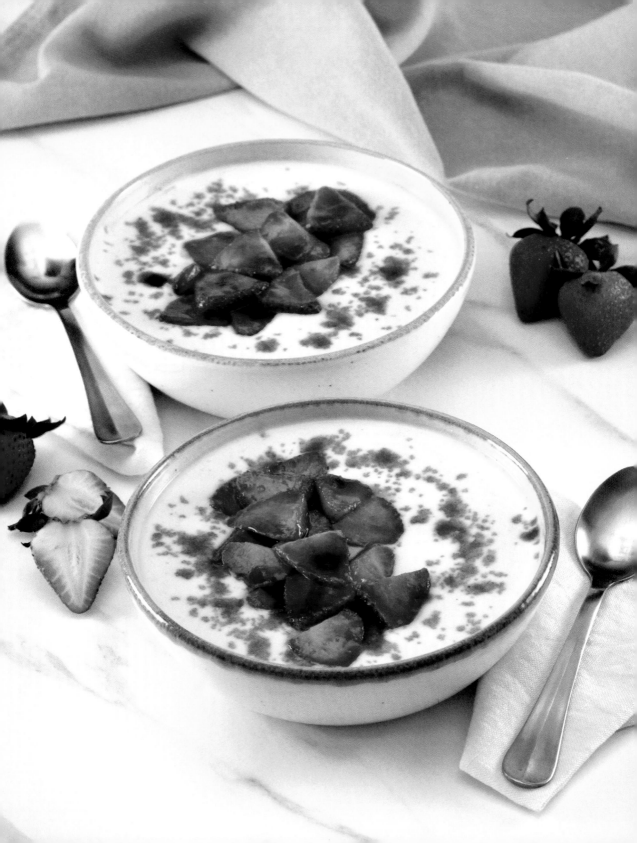

Sautéed Strawberries in Yogurt Soup

Try this dessert when strawberries are in season in your area. You might even be able to cut down on the sugar if your strawberries are already very sweet! To make the most of this delectable dessert, serve with a small scoop of vanilla ice cream.

SERVES 4

1 cup skim milk

1 vanilla bean

2 tablespoons sugar

2 cups plain nonfat yogurt

1 tablespoon unsalted butter

1 pint strawberries, sliced

¼ cup brown sugar

1 Combine milk, vanilla bean, and sugar in a small saucepan over medium heat. Cook for 5 minutes; do not boil. Cool to room temperature and remove vanilla bean. Whisk in yogurt.

2 In a small skillet, melt butter over medium heat. Add strawberries. Sauté, stirring constantly for 5 minutes.

3 Pour yogurt mixture into shallow bowls. Dollop with strawberry mixture and sprinkle with brown sugar and serve.

Calories 190

PER SERVING

Fat 3g
Sodium 115mg
Carbohydrates 34g
Fiber 1g
Sugar 32g
Protein 9g

SUMMER REFRESHMENT

This recipe works well with other summer fruits, such as blackberries, blueberries, raspberries, or ripe peaches. A perfect ending to a picnic, the dessert provides a sweet, light finish to any summer meal.

Almond Biscuits

*Almond (*mygdalota *in Greek) biscuits are a staple product in any Greek bakery. Their light flavor and low calorie count means that you can enjoy them every once in a while, even when you are trying not to overindulge. Refer to step 1 of the Almond Tangerine Bites recipe in this chapter for instructions on blanching almonds.*

SERVES 28

1 pound blanched almonds	3 large eggs, separated and divided	1 tablespoon orange blossom water
1 tablespoon fine semolina flour	1½ cups sugar	28 whole almonds

1 Preheat oven to 350°F. Purée blanched almonds and semolina in food processor until very fine.

2 In a large bowl, beat 2 egg yolks and 1 egg white; add sugar, almond purée, and orange blossom water. Mix well in a stand mixer with a dough hook attachment or by hand with a wooden spoon.

3 In a small mixing bowl, whip 2 egg whites until nice and stiff with peaks; incorporate thoroughly into almond purée.

4 Take up small pieces of dough and roll into balls between palms. Place 28 balls on two large baking sheets lined with parchment paper and press an almond into center of each, flattening lower hemisphere of biscuit.

5 Bake for 20–30 minutes, or until cookies start to turn slightly golden. Remove from oven and let cool at least 1 hour before serving.

6 To maintain the inner chewiness of these biscuits, store in a sealed, airtight container or wrapped in cellophane or plastic.

Calories 150

PER SERVING

Fat 9g
Sodium 10mg
Carbohydrates 14g
Fiber 2g
Sugar 12g
Protein 4g

Cypriot Cookies

This special treat is featured at special events, such as weddings, in Cyprus. You can use any type of marmalade, jam, or preserved fruit for the filling of these cookies.

SERVES 20

8 tablespoons unsalted butter

2 cups all-purpose flour

1$1/2$ cups 2% milk

$1/2$ cup sugar

1 large egg, beaten

1 teaspoon baking powder

$1/2$ cup orange marmalade

1 cup finely chopped almonds

2 tablespoons orange blossom water

$1/2$ teaspoon ground cinnamon

$1/2$ teaspoon ground nutmeg

Confectioners' sugar, for dusting

1 Preheat oven to 350°F.

2 In a large pot, melt butter over medium-high heat. Slowly add flour, stirring constantly with wooden spoon to avoid clumping.

3 Reduce heat to medium-low and slowly add milk. Stir continuously as mixture thickens and starts to clump.

4 When all milk has been added, remove from heat and add sugar, egg, and baking powder; mix well until dough is uniformly smooth.

5 In a small bowl, mix marmalade, almonds, orange blossom water, cinnamon, and nutmeg for filling.

6 Use a rolling pin to spread dough out on a floured surface. Roll dough to uniform thickness of a banana peel. Using a round cookie cutter or a small glass, cut out 20 circles from dough.

7 Place small amount of filling mixture in center of each disc. Fold each disc in half over filling into a half-moon shape; tightly pinch together edges to ensure a good seal.

8 Place cookies on a large buttered baking sheet and bake for 20 minutes. Let stand 30 minutes. Sprinkle cookies with confectioners' sugar before serving.

Calories 170

PER SERVING

Fat 8g
Sodium 15mg
Carbohydrates 22g
Fiber 1g
Sugar 11g
Protein 4g

STANDARD US/METRIC MEASUREMENT CONVERSIONS

VOLUME CONVERSIONS	
US Volume Measure	**Metric Equivalent**
⅛ teaspoon	0.5 milliliter
¼ teaspoon	1 milliliter
½ teaspoon	2 milliliters
1 teaspoon	5 milliliters
½ tablespoon	7 milliliters
1 tablespoon (3 teaspoons)	15 milliliters
2 tablespoons (1 fluid ounce)	30 milliliters
¼ cup (4 tablespoons)	60 milliliters
⅓ cup	90 milliliters
½ cup (4 fluid ounces)	125 milliliters
⅔ cup	160 milliliters
¾ cup (6 fluid ounces)	180 milliliters
1 cup (16 tablespoons)	250 milliliters
1 pint (2 cups)	500 milliliters
1 quart (4 cups)	1 liter (about)

OVEN TEMPERATURE CONVERSIONS	
Degrees Fahrenheit	**Degrees Celsius**
200 degrees F	95 degrees C
250 degrees F	120 degrees C
275 degrees F	135 degrees C
300 degrees F	150 degrees C
325 degrees F	160 degrees C
350 degrees F	180 degrees C
375 degrees F	190 degrees C
400 degrees F	205 degrees C
425 degrees F	220 degrees C
450 degrees F	230 degrees C

WEIGHT CONVERSIONS	
US Weight Measure	**Metric Equivalent**
½ ounce	15 grams
1 ounce	30 grams
2 ounces	60 grams
3 ounces	85 grams
¼ pound (4 ounces)	115 grams
½ pound (8 ounces)	225 grams
¾ pound (12 ounces)	340 grams
1 pound (16 ounces)	454 grams

BAKING PAN SIZES	
American	**Metric**
8 × 1½ inch round baking pan	20 × 4 cm cake tin
9 × 1½ inch round baking pan	23 × 3.5 cm cake tin
11 × 7 × 1½ inch baking pan	28 × 18 × 4 cm baking tin
13 × 9 × 2 inch baking pan	30 × 20 × 5 cm baking tin
2 quart rectangular baking dish	30 × 20 × 3 cm baking tin
15 × 10 × 2 inch baking pan	30 × 25 × 2 cm baking tin (Swiss roll tin)
9 inch pie plate	22 × 4 or 23 × 4 cm pie plate
7 or 8 inch springform pan	18 or 20 cm springform or loose bottom cake tin
9 × 5 × 3 inch loaf pan	23 × 13 × 7 cm or 2 lb narrow loaf or pate tin
1½ quart casserole	1.5 liter casserole
2 quart casserole	2 liter casserole

INDEX